Extracorporeal Shock Wave Lithotripsy

# Extracorporeal Shock Wave Lithotripsy

## Technical Concept, Experimental Research, and Clinical Application

Ch. Chaussy[1], E. Schmiedt, D. Jocham, G. Fuchs[1], W. Brendel
Urological Clinic and Polyclinic and Institute for Surgical Research
of Ludwig-Maximilians-University Munich,
[1]Division of Urology, UCLA School of Medicine, Los Angeles, Calif., USA

B. Forssmann, W. Hepp
Dornier System GmbH, Friedrichshafen

Editor
*Ch. Chaussy,* Munich; Los Angeles, Calif.

81 figures (8 in color) and 25 tables, 1986

2nd, Revised and Enlarged Edition

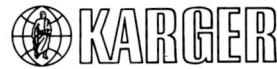

Basel · München · Paris · London · New York · New Delhi · Singapore · Tokyo · Sydney

Title of the original German version: „Berührungsfreie Nierensteinzertrümmerung durch extrakorporal erzeugte, fokussierte Stoßwellen", Beiträge zur Urologie, vol. 2 (Karger, Basel 1980), ISBN 3-8055-1901-X

Section 1-4 of this work was produced by Christian Chaussy, M.D., Professor of Urology of the Medical Faculty of the Ludwig-Maximilians-University, Munich, as habilitation thesis. The research was supported by the Federal Ministry of Research and Technology under Project Designation 01 V1 024-Z13MT 224 a.

Translation into English of Section 1-4 with the help of

Charles Brown and Heike Charest
Gainesville, Florida

National Library of Medicine Cataloging in Publication

Berührungsfreie Nierensteinzertrümmerung durch extrakorporal erzeugte, fokussierte Stoßwellen. English Extracorporeal shock waves lithotripsy: technical concept, experimental research, and clinical application / Ch. Chaussy . . . . [et al.]; editor, Ch. Chaussy; [translation into English with the help of Charles Brown and Heike Charest]. — 2nd rev. and enl. ed. — Basel; New York: Karger, 1986. —

"Produced by Christian Chaussy, M.D., professor of urology of the Medical Faculty of the Ludwig-Maximilians University, Munich, as habilitation thesis. The research was supported by the Federal Ministry of Research and Technology under project designation 01 V1 024-Z13MT 224a"— T.p. verso. Translation of: Berührungsfreie Nierensteinzertrümmerung durch extrakorporal erzeugte, fokussierte Stoßwellen.

Bibliography: p.
ISBN 3-8055-4360-3

1. Kidney Calculi — therapy 2. Lithotripsy I. Chaussy, Ch. (Christian)
II. Germany (West). Bundesministerium für Forschung und Technologie
III. Title

WJ 356 B552

All rights reserved.
No part of this publication may be translated into other languages, reproduced or utilized in any form or by any means, electronic or mechanical, including photocopying, recording, microcopying or by any informations storage and retrieval system, without permission in writing from the publisher.
© Copyright 1986 by S. Karger GmbH, Postfach, D-8034 Germering/München (FRG) and S. Karger AG, P.O. Box, CH-4009 Basel (Switzerland)
Printed in Germany by Ernst Kieser GmbH, D-8902 Neusäß
ISBN 3-8055-4360-3

# Contents

| | |
|---|---|
| *Preface* .................................................. | VIII |
| *Introduction* ............................................ | 1 |
|     Current physical and chemical methods of urinary stone removal .... | 2 |
|     Electrohydraulic shock wave ............................. | 3 |
|     Ultrasonic lithotripsy ................................... | 3 |
|     Shock waves and ultrasound ............................. | 4 |

1. *Shock wave generation, apparatus arrangement, and in vitro testing of the prototype – Methods and results* ...... 7

    1.1   Technical section ................................... 8
    1.1.1 Physical fundamentals ............................ 8
    1.1.2 Shock wave generation and focusing ............... 9

    1.2   Development of the first prototype for the application of shock waves ............................................. 10
    1.2.1 Electrical installation ............................. 10
    1.2.2 Underwater spark gap ........................... 11
    1.2.3 The semi-ellipsoid ............................... 11
    1.2.4 Arrangement of the apparatus ................... 13

    1.3   In vitro testing of the prototype ...................... 13
    1.3.1 Technical pretrials ............................... 13
    1.3.2 Pressure amplitude at varying electrode separation .. 15
    1.3.3 Pressure amplitude at varying discharge voltages .... 15
    1.3.4 Effect of the discharge rate ...................... 15
    1.3.5 Damping and focusing with transmission through tissue ...... 17

    1.4   Summary of the technical trials ...................... 19

2. *In vitro and in vivo studies on biological systems* .................... 21

    2.1   Method ........................................... 22
    2.1.1 In vitro kidney stone destruction – Exposure of urinary stones in a water bath ................... 22
    2.1.2 Photographic studies for the determination of the rate and energy of stone destruction ........................ 22
    2.1.3 Shock wave exposure ............................ 22
    2.1.4 Exposure of lymphocyte cultures .................. 23
    2.1.5 In vivo studies in rats ........................... 24

| | | |
|---|---|---|
| 2.2 | Results | 24 |
| 2.2.1 | Kidney stone destruction in vitro | 24 |
| 2.2.2 | Rate and kinetic energy of stone fragments | 25 |
| 2.2.3 | Evaluation of hemolysis | 33 |
| 2.2.4 | Application of the shock waves to mixed lymphocyte cultures | 34 |
| 2.2.5 | In vivo studies in rats | 34 |
| 2.3 | Evaluation of the pretrial | 35 |

3. *Studies for experimental in vivo stone destruction – Development of an apparatus for experimental in vivo stone destruction* .................. 37

| | | |
|---|---|---|
| 3.1 | Methods | 38 |
| 3.1.1 | Integration of an ultrasonic location system | 38 |
| 3.1.2 | Integration of an ultrasonic B-scanner | 39 |
| 3.1.3 | Experimental apparatus | 41 |
| 3.1.4 | Experimental stone model | 42 |
| 3.1.5 | Animal studies | 43 |
| 3.2 | Results | 44 |
| 3.2.1 | Stone implantation | 44 |
| 3.2.2 | Integration of the ultrasonic location system | 46 |
| 3.2.3 | In vivo studies of stone destruction | 50 |
| 3.3 | Evaluation of the first large animal studies | 56 |

4. *Preclinical shock wave applicator* ................................. 57

| | | |
|---|---|---|
| 4.1 | Methods | 58 |
| 4.1.1 | Prestudies of X-ray location | 58 |
| 4.1.2 | Integration of the X-ray locator | 58 |
| 4.1.3 | Shock wave applicator | 59 |
| 4.1.4 | Changes of the shock wave energy/impulse series | 62 |
| 4.1.5 | Animal studies | 62 |
| 4.2 | Results | 63 |
| 4.2.1 | Effect of intervening water on X-ray location | 63 |
| 4.2.2 | Problems of pseudocavitation | 63 |
| 4.2.3 | Kidney stone destruction with series impulses | 65 |
| 4.2.4 | Chemical studies after in vivo treatments | 65 |
| 4.2.5 | Comparitive clearance studies with $^{99m}$Tc-DMSA | 66 |
| 4.2.6 | Histological evaluation | 68 |
| 4.2.7 | In vivo stone destruction | 68 |

*Discussion* ................................................................. 75

| | |
|---|---|
| The danger of tissue damage | 76 |
| The stone model | 80 |
| Location system | 81 |
| Discharge capability of the concretion fragments | 82 |
| Clinical application and indication | 83 |

*Summary* ................................................................... 87

*Literature* .................................................................. 89

| | | |
|---|---|---|
| 5. | Clinical experience with extracorporeal shock wave lithotripsy (ESWL) | 95 |
| | 5.1   History of the clinical application of ESWL | 96 |
| | 5.2   Indications for ESWL | 99 |
| | 5.2.1 Patient selection | 99 |
| | 5.2.2 Current contraindications | 100 |
| | 5.3   Course of the routine ESWL treatment | 101 |
| | 5.3.1 Patient preparation | 101 |
| | 5.3.2 Anesthesia | 103 |
| | 5.3.3 Shock wave treatment | 104 |
| | 5.3.4 After-care and follow-up | 110 |
| | 5.4   ESWL management of urinary stones | 112 |
| | 5.4.1 Treatment of pelvic and caliceal stones < 2.5 cm | 112 |
| | 5.4.2 Treatment of staghorn stones | 112 |
| | 5.4.3 Treatment of ureteral stones | 125 |
| | 5.4.4 Treatment of infected stones | 136 |
| | 5.4.5 Treatment of radiolucent and semi-opaque stones | 137 |
| | 5.4.6 Treatment of bilateral stones | 139 |
| | 5.4.7 Treatment of children | 139 |
| | 5.4.8 Treatment of medical risk group patients | 141 |
| | 5.4.9 Treatment of stones with distal obstruction | 142 |
| | 5.4.10 Treatment of the "inoperable" stone | 142 |
| | 5.5   Results of ESWL therapy | 143 |
| | 5.5.1 Renal function | 144 |
| | 5.5.2 Complications of ESWL and management of ESWL-related complications | 145 |
| | 5.6   The role of ESWL in current concepts of urinary stone management | 150 |
| Literature | | 154 |

# Preface

Slightly more than 4 years have passed since the first edition of this book on extracorporeal shock wave lithotripsy (ESWL) was introduced. During this relatively short period of time, noninvasive means of disintegrating human urinary stones have completely changed the management of urinary stone disease. Today ESWL has proven its safety, efficacy and reliability. This has been demonstrated by the steadily increasing number of lithotripter facilities all over the world and the more than 100,000 successfully performed treatments. Due to its high success rate and the absence of severe complications, ESWL has almost completely surplanted open surgical, and to a lesser extent endourological procedures. The reason for this surprisingly rapid progress with this new methodology can be only partially explained by the excellent research cooperation of urologists and physicists. The high demand for a less invasive treatment modality exerted by the stonebearing patients themselves was also a major contributing factor. However, the high expectations of these patients could not be met immediately. It was, at this point, important for the future of this method that the outside pressure did not influence our cautions approach to increase its indications. Based on the noninvasive concept of the methodology a stepwise enlargement of the indications backed by reproducible results was pursued. This finally led to well established indications for the treatment of all upper urinary stones.
We do not know for sure, whether or not we have reached the endpoint of the development of this method and its clinical applications for the treatment of urinary stone disease.
However, it is certain that the progress made by urologists, for the sake of urology, represents a dramatic change in the management of urinary stones by which invasive approaches have been superseded by a noninvasive procedure. From now on all other methods employed for the treatment of urinary stones will have to be judged against the results of this methodology.

Christian G. Chaussy

Los Angeles, Calif., March 1986

# Introduction

In modern surgical practice the purely operative procedures are being increasingly supplemented through the development of new technology. For example, laser techniques in special applications in ophthalmology [48], in gastrointestinal surgery [55, 56, 95] and urology [85] have partially displaced the "therapy with the knife", thus opening new therapeutic possibilities [67].

It may be assumed that medicine is only at the beginning of this development in which the surgeon, through new technological "assistants in hand" working in combination with surgical procedures, finds possible a more discriminating and less risky therapy. The studies presented here are an example of this development.

Attempts to integrate advances in the physical and chemical areas into the therapy of kidney stone disease go far back [2, 84]. Nevertheless operative removal of concretions in the upper urinary tract remains the therapy of choice with only a few exceptions which will be detailed later.

With a morbidity rate of about three percent of urolithiasis cases in the total population of the Federal Republic of Germany [2, 82], there appears to be wide application for the non-invasive method of handling urinary stone disease. A segment of stone-carrying patients never show any symptoms and are never diagnosed and approximately 80 % of kidney stones are discharged spontaneously [9, 10, 17, 99], yet surgical removal remains the most frequent course of surgical assistance in the urological clinic.

The quantity of these surgical stone removals provides a motivation for a new, alternative, non-invasive method of stone destruction. But it is surprising that regarding the quantity of these surgical stone removals, no statistics have been compiled in the Federal Republic either on a national level or a state level.

Therefore in cooperation with the statisticians of Dornier System a survey was conducted at 80 randomly selected urology clinics.

Table I repeats the salient points of the questionnaire. It shows a total of 49,750 urinary stone removals of which 35.8 % were kidney stone removals.

*Table I.* Totals of operations performed in 1976 in 358 urological clinics and hospitals in the Federal Republic of Germany for the removal or urinary stones

| Total of all operations | 49,750 | |
|---|---|---|
| | Subtotals | % |
| Kidney stones | 17,800 | 35.8 |
| Ureter stones | 20,420 | 41.0 |
| Bladder stones | 5,940 | 12.0 |
| Urinary stone removals with surgery (i.e. Zeiss sling, lithotripsy) | 5,590 | 11.2 |

An interesting revelation of these statistics is that in 11.2 % of the cases the stones were freed by a transurethral procedure without surgery.

The purpose of the presented work is to develop a procedure for the contact-free destruction of kidney stones using new physical methods.

*Current physical and chemical methods of urinary stone removal*

The only currently available, practicable, non-invasive therapy for urinary stone disease is chemotherapy for uric acid stones [5, 44, 60, 61]. In this therapy, through the alkalizing of the urine, the existing stone is dissolved and, in most cases, the patient is cured of his disease. However, sometimes the patient's condition is already so acute that immediate surgery is imperative. For example, when a stone has blocked the ureter and the urine has become infected, the threatening urosepsis prohibits waiting for weeks while chemotherapy takes effect [44, 61].

Attempts at chemical dissolution of all other types of stone, with very few exceptions, have failed [1, 94]. On the one hand, an irrigation technique that had been successful in vitro resulted in nephrotoxicity and, on the other hand, the irrigation device placed in the kidney cavity requiring the months-long immobilization of the patient [9, 71] was found to increase the chance of stone formation in the untreated kidney. Besides, the high complication rate from the irrigation device because of increasing infection with the buildup of urosepsis indicates that neither of these methods will find a place in the routine treatment of kidney stone patients [1, 9, 71].

Although limited in application, the currently practiced physical methods of stone destruction have proven more successful. All these methods have in common that they necessitate the direct contact of the concretion and the energy source. Therefore they are all either transurethral or surgical. To name two, there are the electrohydraulic shock wave and the ultrasonic lithotripter.

*Electrohydraulic shock wave*

Two well-isolated, high voltage leads are carried by a common cystoscope with a working attachment to the stone. A high capacity condenser is discharged via this probe, whereby a spark jumps between two poles, an axial and a cylindrical electrode at the tip of the probe. Through this sparking, a hydrodynamic wave is created which destroys the concretion upon contact [16, 30, 36]. Today, this method is a routine form of treatment for bladder stones [57, 58].

*Ultrasonic lithotripsy*

Ultrasonic waves (27,000/sec) are produced by an ultrasonic generator. High frequency electrical energy is transformed into mechanical energy by an ultrasound converter and carried by a hollow steel probe, which in turn conveys the energy to the concretion [73, 74, 63]. This also requires a contact between the probe and the concretion so that application with the cystoscope is limited to bladder stones [88, 89, 90, 91].

For both methods, experimental studies are presently being conducted to miniaturize the apparatus with the goal of extending its application to ureter stones [53, 70, 73, 83]. In each case, optical control of the probe-stone contact is required for riskless application. Integration of the optical system, the irrigation canal and the working probe with a diameter of about 3 mm for application in the ureter has not yet been solved satisfactorily [30, 36, 70, 74]. In addition it is known from experience with bladder stone lithotripsy that there has to be a distance between the probe and the bladder wall of three to five millimeters. With closer contact there is the danger of bladder wall lesions or perhaps even perforation [62, 92]. This "safety intervall" cannot be achieved in the ureter so that with the currently available probes there is a danger of ureter damage and perforation [30, 36, 74].

Studies by Forster and Thammen revealed that ureter soundings, even under sterile conditions, result in approximately 20 % of patients acquiring urinary tract infection [34]. The same value must also be applied to probe lithotripsy of ureter stones. With the consequent appearance of a hindrance of flow in the urinary tract following stone destruction and the occurence of infection, a high post-operative complication rate may be counted upon.

Surely part of this problem will be solved through new discoveries, and one of these methods, when specially indicated, can become an alternative to surgical removal of urinary stones. But it still remains that both methods require invasive operative (transurethral) procedures, and therefore an externally applied method such as the shock wave technique presented here is motivated.


*Shock waves and ultrasound*

New results in the area of high-speed physics [26, 39, 41] have opened the possibility of contact-free destruction of concretions by the application of high energy shock waves from a distance [40, 42, 47]. The first in vitro successes [39] were accomplished with shock waves which were created by impact of high speed projectiles or the elastic impulse of a detonating wire [42]. Indeed, at the beginning, there was no acceptable means of generating such waves as required for clinical use.

Only after the development of a method of generating shock waves by the underwater spark gap [6, 7, 32, 43, 59, 69] were the technical and application requirements met so that studies could be undertaken with the goal of clinical applications [19-23, 27-29].

At the time that physical findings suggested the external application of shock waves as a treatment for urinary stone disease (Patent 2351247), the only information available related to the action of these waves on brittle materials [43, 68]. There certainly was no recourse to information on application to biological structures. On the other hand, there are numerous studies related to the effects of ultrasound in medicine [45, 63, 64, 65, 76]. Although the physical laws of acoustics apply to both wave forms, there are great differences in the physical and energetic properties of ultrasound and shock waves.

When the pressure vs. time diagrams of ultrasound and shock waves are compared, it is seen that a shock wave has a single pressure spike with very steep onset and gradual relaxation. On the other hand the ultrasonic wave has a sinusoidal pressure variation with an alternating tension and compression [32].

In addition, shock waves and ultrasound have a different frequency spectrum. While the ultrasonic wave has a well-defined frequency, the shock wave has a spectrum composed of both low and high frequencies. The effect of both waves can be observed as they are dissipated during transmission through materials.

In principle, it can be said that by transmission through biological materials, high frequency parts of the wave are much more effectively damped than the low frequency portions [37, 50]. This results in significantly less damping of the shock wave, which has an extensive low frequency range in comparison with the ultrasound [49]. Therefore the depth of penetration of the shock waves is greater than that of the ultrasound.

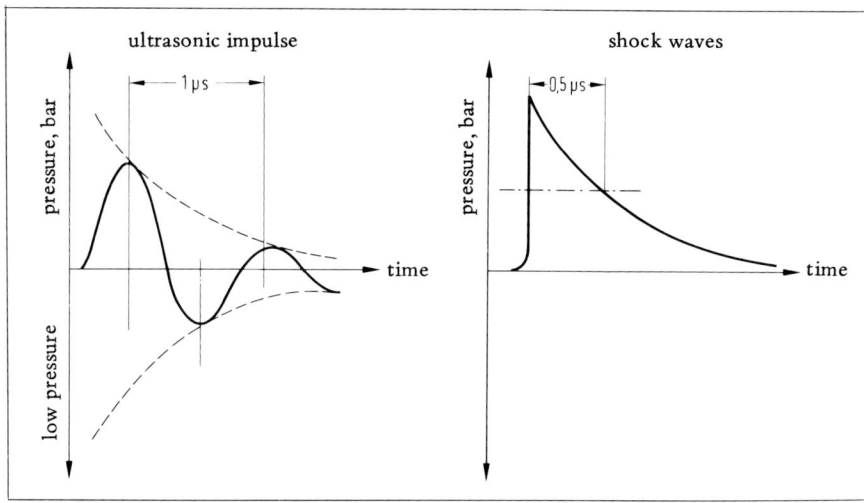

*Figure 1.* Comparison of the pressure vs. time diagrams for ultrasound and a shock wave.

Because of the strong damping effect during transmission in materials, long exposure to ultrasound results in cellular degradation; based on this absorption effect this can be best explained as a thermal degradation [27, 64, 65]. Even at high energies, such lesions do not occur from shock wave exposure.

With the shock wave technique on biological systems, genuinely new territory had been entered. Therefore the need arose to do basic studies of the effect of such high energy waves on cellular structures before approaching the task of developing the technique for the external application of shock waves as a means for the destruction of kidney stones.

In addition, there was a need to develop the necessary accessories for application of the shock wave device which made possible experimental studies on preclinical models. These innovations were the result of actual studies conducted on animals as opposed to technical or physical requirements.

As a result of these studies different developmental steps were tried, which after review of the experimental results led to either changes or additions to the construction of the shock wave device.

Corresponding with these developmental steps, the here presented work falls into five parts, where after the introduction to the basic apparatus and the experimental pretrials, the second part presents the first in vivo and in vitro trials. In the third part are presented in vivo studies of experimental stone destruction conducted with the altered apparatus. Through the development, as a consequence of phase three, of preclinical shock wave devices, a new conception of the experimental apparatus was developed, which is described along with the animal studies in part four. Part 5 summarizes the first clinical experience with extracorporeal shock wave lithotripsy.

Consequently, descriptions of methods, apparatus, and experimental procedure are found in the appropriate sections.

# 1. Shock wave generation, apparatus arrangement, and in vitro testing of the prototype- methods and results

## 1.1 Technical section

### 1.1.1 Physical fundamentals

When the pressure wave comes in contact with an interface, the sound impedance changes, so that the compression phase or tensile phase is reflected depending on the acoustical quality of this interface. At the point where the pressure wave exceeds the strength of the material, mechanical destruction occurs. This theoretical physical definition given by R. *Schall* [81] provides a useful basis for the destruction of kidney stones.

This destruction process can be shown schematically by the following simple model (figure 2):

An externally generated shock wave enters the body and propagates without interference because there is virtually no difference in acoustic impedance between body tissues and water [42]. At the tissue/concretion interface, by partial reflection of the shock wave, a high pressure load is established, which destroys the concretion in the region of zone A. The transmitted wave is reflected at the opposite side with a phase reversal so that it becomes a tensile wave [75]. Destruction in zone B is accomplished when the limit of tensile strength is exceeded. The unaffected zone C must be subjected to another exposure. The depth of an individual destruction zone and the degree of destruction depend very decisively on the intensity of the pressure amplitude and the length of the impulse.

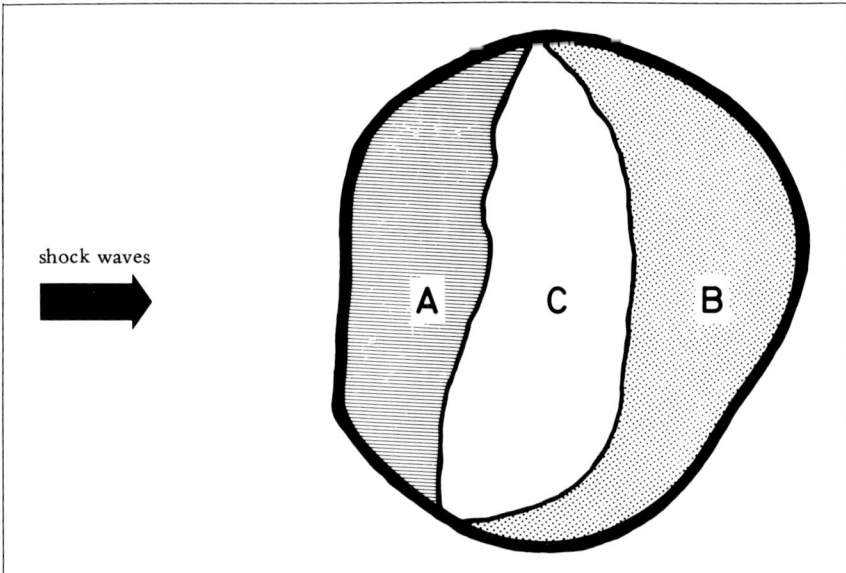

*Figure 2.* Schematic description of stone destruction.

To accomplish the reduction of concretions in biological tissues, five requirements must be fulfilled:

1. The pressure amplitude of the shock wave must greatly exceed the compressive and tensile strength of the stone.

2. The necessary pressure amplitude for stone destruction must lie below the tolerance level of biological tissues.

3. In order to take advantage of the splitting-off effect in overcoming the tensile strength, the length of the impulse of the shock wave must be shorter than the transit time through the kidney stone so that the superposition of the entering and reflected waves will be avoided, this means that the time extent of the pressure shock must be in the order of microseconds.

4. A focusing of the shock wave must be striven after in order to avoid stress on tissue as much as possible. In this way, the maximum pressure amplitude is achieved at the focus while at points away from the focus there is a greatly reduced pressure stress.

5. In order to avoid harmful reflection and the resulting stress on the body surface, the shock wave must be introduced into the body in a medium where the sonic impedance is similar to the sonic impedance of biological tissues.

*1.1.2 Shock wave generation and focusing*

In all experiments the shock waves are produced by an underwater spark discharge. By this means, the energy stored in a condenser is released in a very short time. Thereby, an arc arises between the electrodes which, in approximately 1 microsecond, vaporizes the fluid surrounding the arc's path, establishing a plasma-like state. The result is an explosionlike vaporization of the fluid. Because of the rapid evaporation a shock wave is created in the surrounding fluid which spreads out in a circular fashion.

The focusing of the shock wave is accomplished thus: A shock wave is generated at the focal point (f 1) of a rotationally symmetrical semi-ellipsoid, it is reflected off the elliptical wall and concentrates at the second focal point (f 2).

The focusing of such an ellipse is explained in the following manner: After being generated, the shock wave spreads in a circular form until it reaches the ellipsoid wall. Each point of the ellispoid wall becomes a generating point for a new circular wave. The reflected shock wave front forms the envelope of these elementary waves.

In figure 3, these wave front envelopes are sketched as they appear at different times. With increasing time the waves move toward the right until they convene at the second focal point (f 2). The focusing effect of the ellipsoid leads to clearly definable transmission time because all the shock waves which are reflected from the ellipsoid wall convene at the objective focal point.

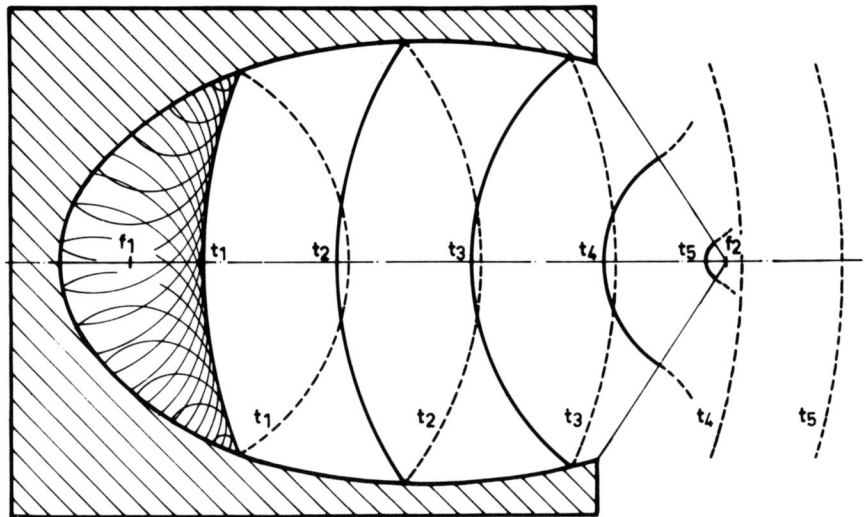

*Figure 3.* Propagation/time diagram of a shock wave expanding from the first focal point (f1) of the semi-ellipsoid (f2=second focal point and the focus of the ellipsoid).

## 1.2 Development of the first prototype for the application of shock waves

### 1.2.1 Electrical installation

In the first experimental model a condenser battery with a capacitance of 1.25 microfarads and a voltage of 40 kV was employed. The maximum energy realized from this arrangement was 560 joules. In order to establish the steepest possible current onset, the inductance of the circuit had to be kept small. As is shown in the schematic circuit diagram (figure 4), the entire inductance is the

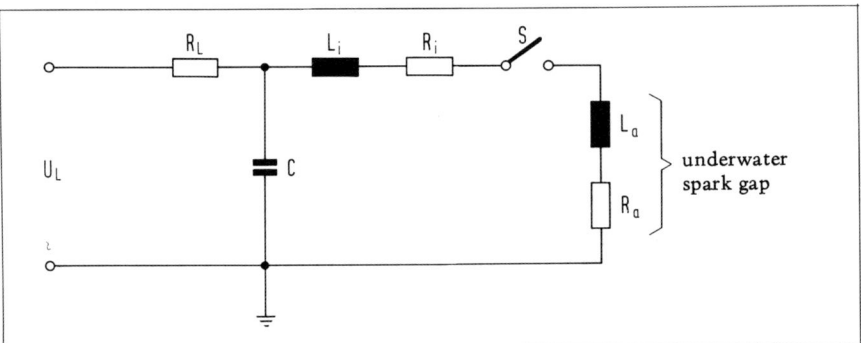

*Figure 4.* Equivalent circuit diagram. $U_L$: charging voltage, $R_L$: charge resistance, C: condenser, $L_i$: inner inductivity, $R_i$: inner resistance, $R_a$: load resistance, S: circuit spark gap, $L_a$: outer inductivity.

*Table II.* Technical data on the first experimental model for the application of shock waves

| | |
|---|---|
| Operating voltage | 27 kV |
| Condenser capacitance | 2 microFarad |
| Impulse duration | 1 microsecond |
| Pressure amplitude | about 1.5 kbar |
| Speed of propagation of the shock wave | 1500 m/sec |

sum of the inner inductance of the discharge circuit ($L_i$) and an outer inductance of the spark gap ($L_a$).

The inner inductance of the discharge circuit arises from the internal inductance of the condenser and from the inductance of the leads. In order to achieve the highest possible current, the condenser must discharge very quickly. This cannot be achieved by a mechanical switch. Therefore, an electrode spark gap (S) with a very low ignition time [32] must be employed as a switch. It can fire at 40 % of the breakthrough voltage.

The electrical data of the shock wave generator are presented in table II.

### 1.2.2 Underwater spark gap

The following requirements are established for the underwater spark gap:

1. Low inductance
2. Extremely high mechanical strength
3. No disturbing of the spreading of the shock wave.

For the elctrodes, steel rods 4 mm in diameter were employed, having tungsten tips with a taper of 25° (figure 5).

The steel rods were isolated from the rest of the device by a synthetic material. The electrode separation can be altered up to a maximum of 55mm. The high mechanical stress, which occurs at generation of the shock wave, is taken into account by the elasticity of the electrode tips. The electrode tips spread apart during each firing and close back to their rest position immediately afterwards. Nevertheless, the lifetime of the underwater spark gap remains limited to 50-100 uses because local overheating of the electrode tip during the discharge cycle erodes the material of the electrode.

### 1.2.3 The semi-ellipsoid

In order to focus the shock waves a rotationally symmetrical reflector was manufactured from brass (figure 6).

The maximum semi-axis was 11 cm and the minimum semi-axis was 6.5 cm. Through a hole bored in the side the electrode system can be positioned at the focal point of the ellipsoid. Water was used as filling fluid. The reflector is in-

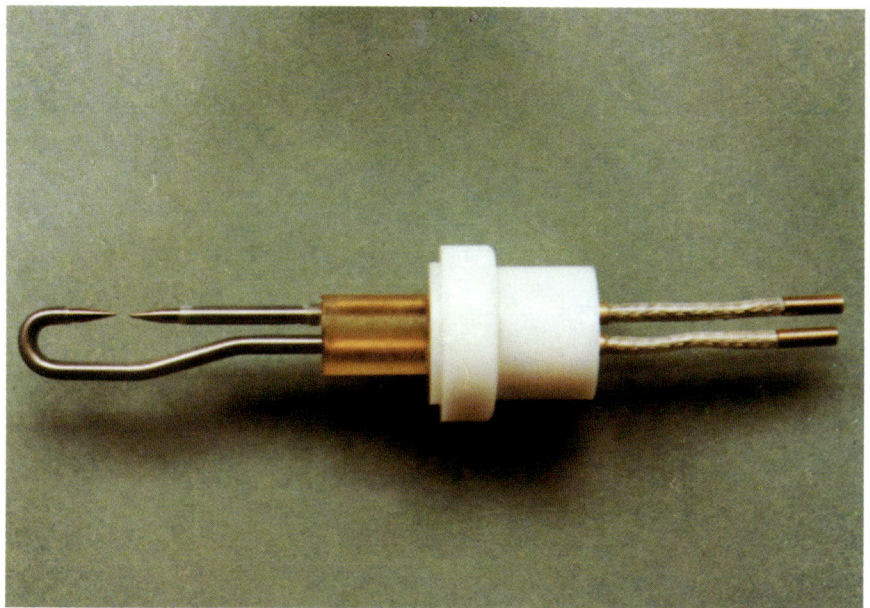

*Figure 5.* Detailed picture of the arrangement of the electrodes of the underwater spark gap (scale: ca. 50 % of natural size).

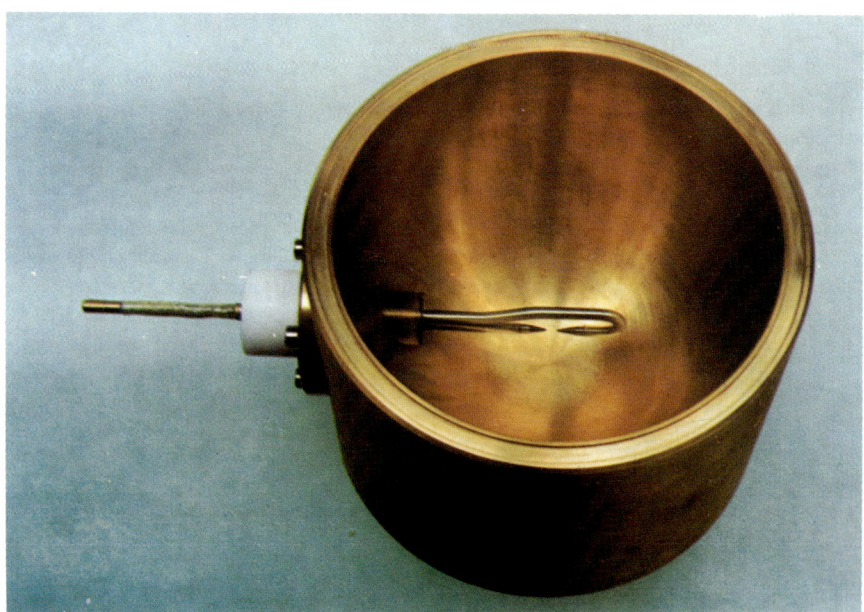

*Figure 6.* Shock wave reflector with electrode entering from side.

sulated with a 0,3 mm thick polyurethane sheet so that the electrical portion of the device is separated from the trial area.

### 1.2.4 Arrangement of the apparatus

Figure 7 shows the completed assembly of the previously described individual parts. On the left side of the apparatus the electrical portions are found and on the right is the ellipsoid equipped experimental bath in which the first in vitro and in vivo trials were conducted. Water was used as the coupling medium.

This experimental tub could be exchanged with a table lying in the focal plane.

## 1.3 In vitro testing of the prototype

### 1.3.1 Technical pretrials

The pressure amplitude of the shock wave could in principle be influenced by a change of the charge on the condenser or through a change of the electrode separation thus influencing the discharge width of the underwater spark.

Studies were conducted to verify these parameters in a trial arrangement shown in figure 8.

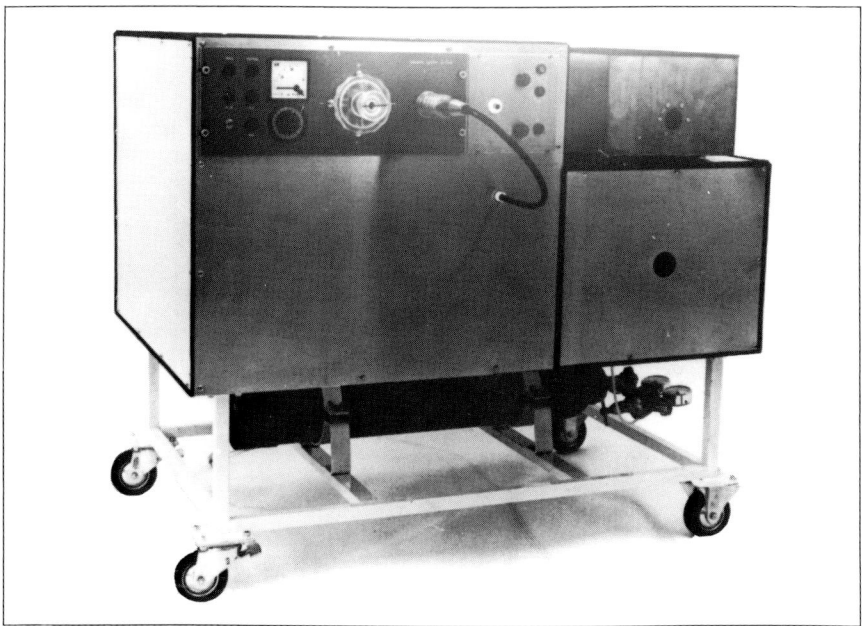

*Figure 7.* Experimental type 1.

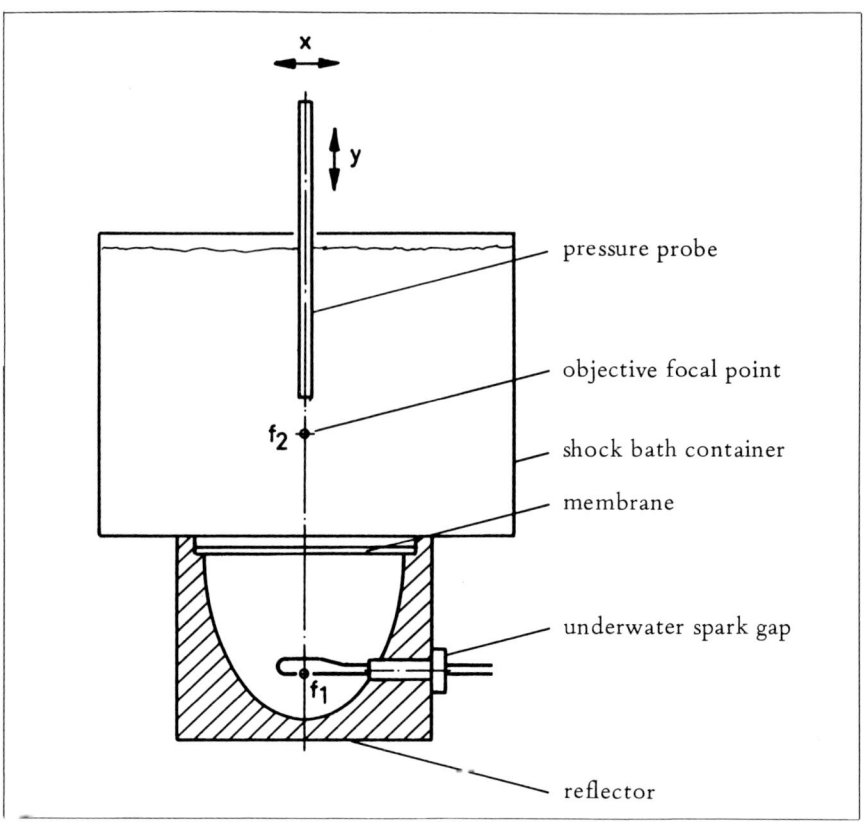

*Figure 8.* Trial arrangement for determination of the pressure amplitude of the shock waves at the second focal point (f 2) of the semi-ellipsoid.

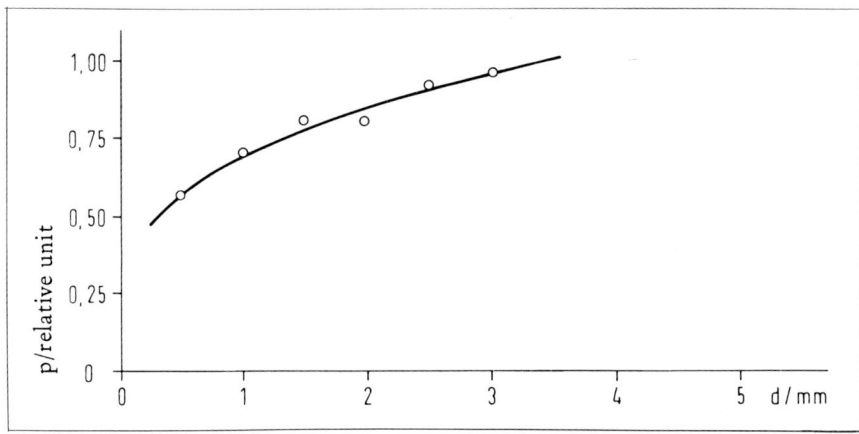

*Figure 9.* Dependence of the shock wave intensity, p, on the underwater spark gap electrode separation, d.

To this end the first prototype whose construction is described was employed, and a piezoelectric pressure probe was positioned at the focal point of the ellipsoid.

*1.3.2 Pressure amplitude at varying electrode separation*

By changing the electrode separation in the range of 0.5-3.5 mm the dependence of the pressure amplitude on the separation of the electrodes could be measured with this experimental arrangement. During these experiments the condenser charge was held constant at 15 kV.

As is shown in figure 9, an increase in the electrode separation appears as an increased pressure amplitude on the objective side. The pressure amplitude was almost doubled by an increase in the electrode separation from 1 mm to 3.5 mm.

With a longer discharge gap there is an increase in the passage created by the plasma, resulting in a greater total energy of the plasma. In this way an increased amount of electrical energy is converted into mechanical energy.

*1.3.3 Pressure amplitude at varying discharge voltages*

With the same experimental arrangement at constant electrode separation, the value of the pressure was measured at different discharge voltages of the condenser.

The energy of the passage created by the plasma is dependent on the energy of the condenser so that a direct proportionality between the discharge voltage and the pressure amplitude is expected.

As the values in figure 10 show, this is only true for the higher voltages. Up to 11 kV no shock wave is generated because the field strength is insufficient to strike an arc on the underwater spark gap. Above this voltage, increasing discharge voltage gives a steep rise in the pressure amplitude which approaches asymptotically a maximum value at voltages exceeding 30 kV.

*1.3.4 Effect of the discharge rate*

With constant electrode separation and unchanged discharge voltage (17.5 kV), the discharge rate was changed through changes in the frequency of the oscillating circuit.

In figure 11, the effect of the oscillating frequency of the discharge circuit on the shock wave duration and the shock wave intensity is shown.

While the duration of the shock wave is independent of the rate of the discharge, there is a pronounced dependency of the intensity of the shock wave on the discharge frequency. With an elevation of the discharge rate there is a rise in the shock wave intensity.

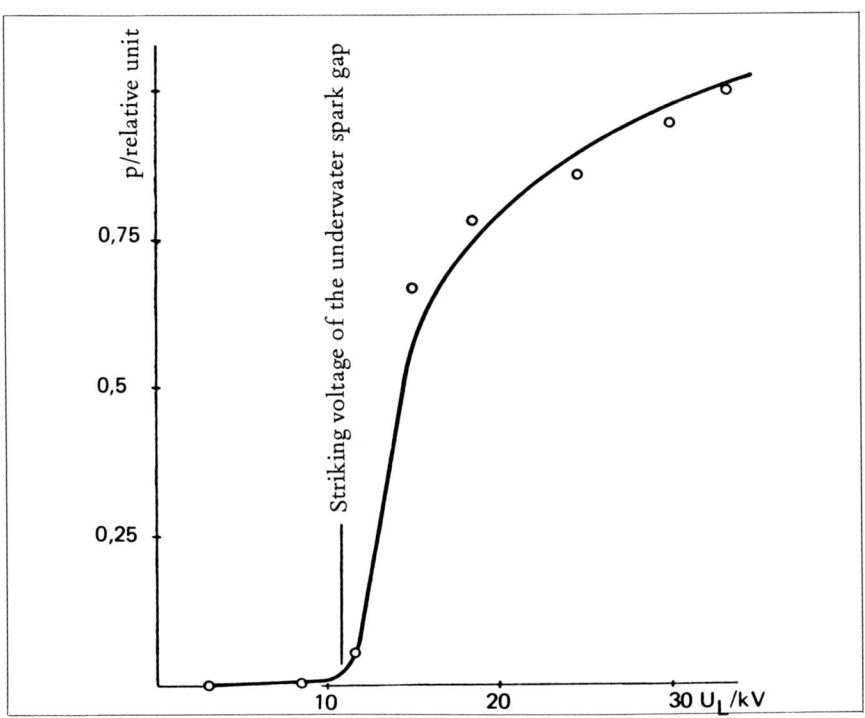

*Figure 10.* Pressure amplitude at the objective focus in dependence on the discharge voltage ($U_L$) of the condenser.

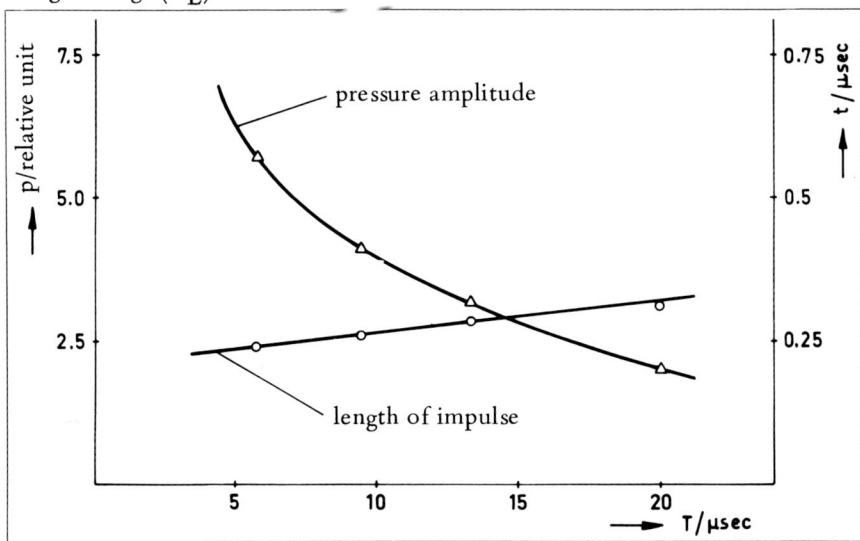

*Figure 11.* Behavior of the shock wave intensity (p) and duration (t) with changing discharge rate of the oscillating circuit.

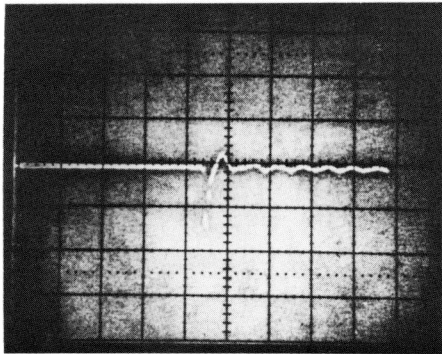

*Figure 12.* Pressure/time diagram of a shock wave at the objective focus. Horizontal scale: 2 microseconds per division. Vertical scale: 5 volts per division.

In figure 12 the pressure time diagram of a shock wave with a discharge rate of 5.5 microseconds is shown. Notice the steep pressure onset of the wavefront. The impulse length, measured at the point where the pressure had dropped by half, is 0.4 microsecond.

*1.3.5 Damping and focusing with transmission through tissue*

In studying the in vivo destruction of kidney stones it is impossible to avoid the transmission of the shock wave through tissue. The pretrials clarified the effect on the profile of the shock wave caused by entry into and transmission through the tissue. In order to study this effect the only change made in the trial apparatus was to position layers of different tissues between the shock wave source and the objective focal point.

These studies revealed a defocusing of the shock waves by interpolated tissue by the discontinuity at the water-tissue interface. The extent of the damping of the pressure amplitude by tissue transmission was also measured.

To accomplish this, a 6 cm thick layer of muscle tissue or a 4 cm thick layer of fatty tissue was inserted. Figure 13 gives the pressure variation of the shock wave on the horizontal axis (ordinate) and on the rotational axis (abscissa) as it passes through the 4 cm layer of fatty tissue.

It was shown that the transmission of a shock wave through biological tissue does not affect the focusing of the elliptical reflector.

To evaluate the damping effect of a shock wave, measurements with a firmly installed pressure probe were conducted with and without interposed tissue. The difference in the maximum amplitude of the shock wave in the control measurement without the tissue and the measurement with the tissue was used as a norm for the damping caused by the tissue.

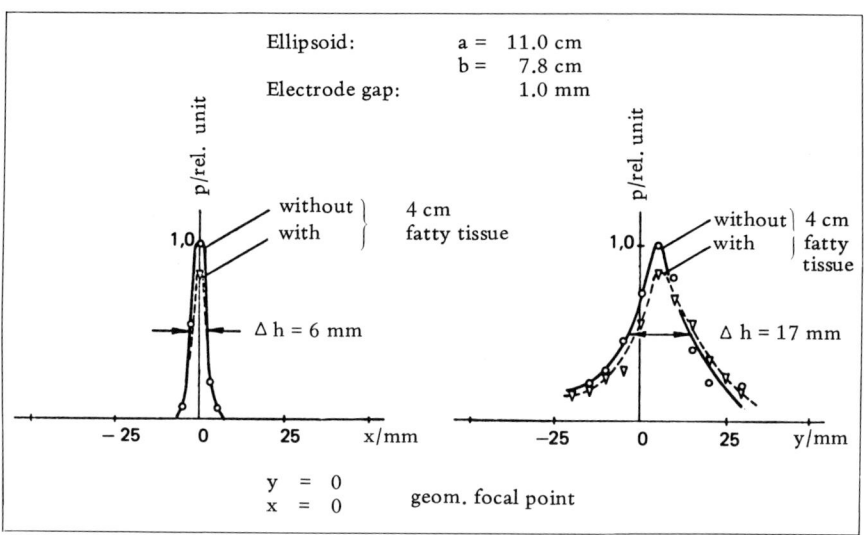

*Figure 13.* Focusing of the shock wave with (circles) and without (triangles) interposed tissue (4 cm fatty tissue) on the rotational axis (abscissa) and on the horizontal axis (ordinate) of the ellipsoid. Pressure amplitude in p.

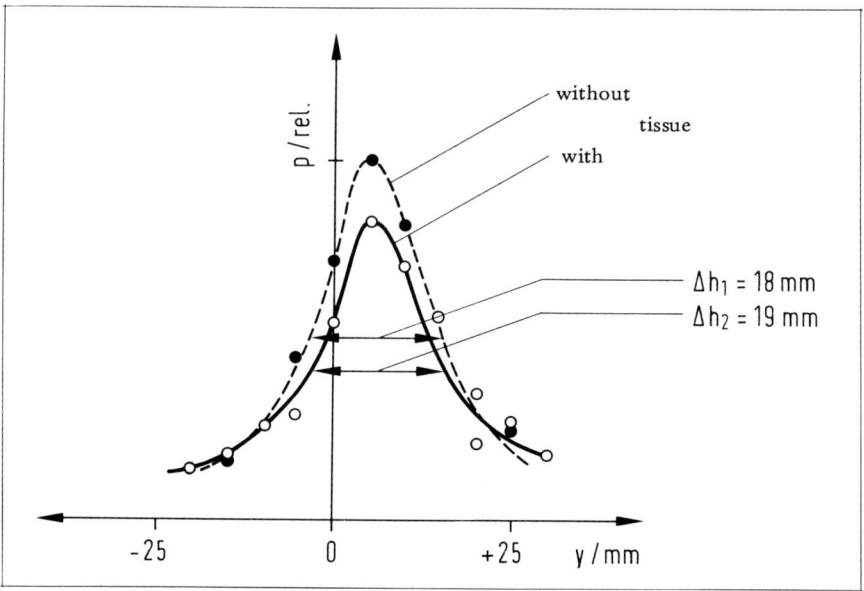

*Figure 14.* Change in pressure amplitude (p) by transmission through a layer of tissue (6 cm muscle).

Figure 14 gives an example of the diminishing of the pressure amplitude by transmission through tissue.

It is shown that with transmission through 6 cm of muscle tissue there is a 10-20% drop in pressure amplitude. The reduction can be compensated by an increase in the pressure amplitude of the shock wave, for example by raising the condenser discharge voltage.

## 1.4 Summary of the technical trials

1. A change or heigthening of the pressure amplitude of the shock wave can be accomplished through widening the electrode separation or increasing the condenser discharge voltage.
   For the experimental type 1, a standard for the modification of the condenser discharge voltage was established at the widest electrode separation (3-5 mm). By this, a condenser voltage of up to 27 kV was possible. At discharge this resulted in a maximum pressure at the second focal point of the ellipse of 3.5 kbar.
2. The transmission measurements show a pronounced correlation between the discharge rate of the switching circuit and the shock wave intensity. The shorter the discharge rate, the higher the shock wave intensity while the duration of the shock wave is unchanged. The discharge rate could be reduced to about 1 microsecond.
3. Interposition of layers of tissue between the first and second focal point of the ellipsoid does not influence the focusing of the shock wave.
4. A damping of the pressure amplitude by transmission through the tissue may be counted upon. By in vitro studies a decrease in the amplitude of 10-20 % was realized for a transmission distance simulating the distance between the body surface and the kidney cavity. This decrease in amplitude can be compensated by an increase in charge on the condenser.

## 2. In vitro and in vivo studies on biological systems

After it became possible to concentrate high energy shock waves in a focus zone of 1.5 cm$^3$, the next objective was in vitro studies to determine if these energies were sufficient to reproducibly reduce urinary stones of different chemical compositions. At the same time it was necessary to determine whether or not energies of this order would have any effect on vital tissue structures.

## 2.1 Method

### 2.1.1 In vitro kidney stone destruction – Exposure of urinary stones in a water bath

Uric acid, calcium oxalate and magnesium ammonium phosphate stones were positioned in the focus zone of the shock waves freely suspended in a water-filled plastic bag (figure 15). Fifty kidney stones of different weights (0.03-14.11 g) were subjected to a maximum of five exposures. The electrode separation of the underwater spark gap was 3.5 mm. The discharge voltage was 27 kV.

### 2.1.2 Photographic studies for the determination of the rate and energy of stone destruction

a) Still photography

The crumbling of the kidney stone was photographed with a flashlamp (Nanolite, Driver, Impulsphysik GmbH, Hamburg-Rissen; T = 20 nsec) in direct light. The time between release of the shock wave and discharge of the flashlamp was varied little by little. The three-dimensional process of stone destruction was projected on a screen.

b) Motion photography

A high speed camera (High-Cam, Weinberger Co., Zurich; maximum of 1,000 frames/second) was used to accomplish photographic analysis of stone destruction. It is possible to estimate the kinetic energy of the individual particles by measuring the distance and speed (taken from successive frames) after the stone destruction.

### 2.1.3 Shock wave exposure

A standard volume of 10 ml of full dog blood (Hemocrit 45 ± 1.5), collected in an air-free tube, was placed in the water bath at the focal point of the ellipsoid.

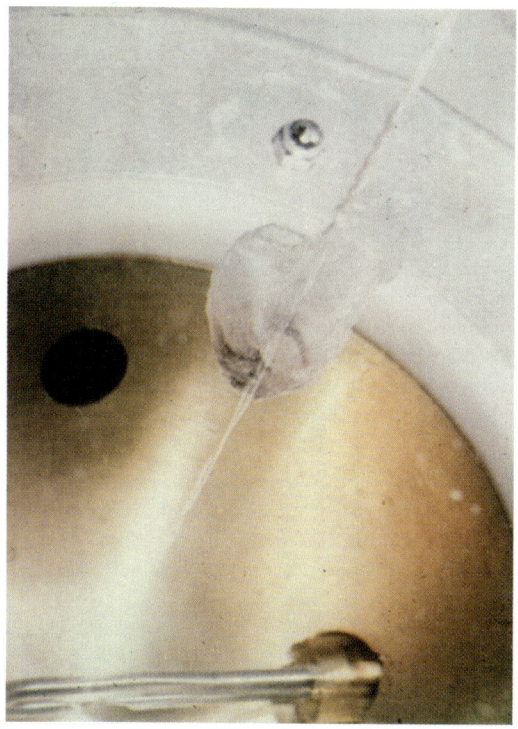

*Figure 15.* Experimental configuration for in vitro urinary stone destruction.

After exposure the blood sample was centrifugated and the free plasma hemoglobin was determined by the cyanogen-hemoglobin method.

The influence of the shock waves was studied on 65 individual samples which had been exposed from 1 to 4 times at an energy of 27 kV. The capability of the instrument was tested before and after each experimental series of shock wave exposures of urinary stones.

### 2.1.4 *Exposure of lymphocyte cultures*

10 ml of full human blood containing heparin were separated with a Ficoll-Isopaque, the lymphocyte fraction was removed and the cells were washed three times with culture medium. Lymphocytes ($12 \times 10^6$ cells) were suspended in 8 ml of medium and divided into four aliquots. Two of the aliquots each containing $1.5 \times 10^6$/ml cells were used as stimulator cells and bombarded with 1500 roentgens.

Equal numbers of bombarded and unbombarded (stimulator and responder) cells were placed in the focus zone. Both the treated and untreated samples were used for mixed lymphocyte culture (MLC) and PHA-culture. After incubation, the cells were labeled with $^3$H-thymidine, precipitated and the resulting activity measured with a scintillation counter.

*2.1.5  In vivo studies in rats*

a) General exposure of the abdominal and thoracic cavities

250 g male Sprague-Dawley rats were anesthetized with 2.5 ml of 3.6 % chloral hydrate and after complete epilation of the abdomen and thorax, they were fixed in the membranous experimental area and thus in the focus zone. The research animals received either 5 or 10 exposures of constant intensity (27 kV, electrode separation = 3.5 mm). In one group the exposure of the thoracic cavity was direct and in a second group a shield of styrofoam was used (5x10x0.3 cm).

After shock wave exposure of the abdominal region, macroscopic tissue samples from the liver, kidney, small intestine, large intestine and spinal column were collected for histological studies. The examination in group 1 (n = 20) was conducted after 24 hours and in group 2 (n = 20), after the rats had lived 14 days.

b) Specific exposure of eventrated organs

After median laparotomy the liver and the intestine were eventrated and placed in the experimental field in the focus zone (figure 16).

These organs were embedded in vaseline on the coupling membrane so that the continuity of the shock wave propagation might not be interrupted by residual air adhering to the surface of the organ. After exposure the organs were replaced, the laparotomy was closed and the animals were put under a controlled environment in cages. Corresponding to the previous procedure, histological samples were collected 24 hours and 14 days after the experiment.

## 2.2  Results

*2.2.1  Kidney stone destruction in vitro*

In the selected trial procedure each urinary stone which was placed in the focus was disintegrated regardless of size or chemical composition. In each case a single shock wave exposure was sufficient to break apart the stone structure and to create several individual parts. Additional shock wave exposure brought about more destruction and disintegration of the individual fragments. In concretions where the diameter was greater than the selected focus zone of 1.5 cm, adjustments were necessary in order to complete the treatment of outlying fragments.

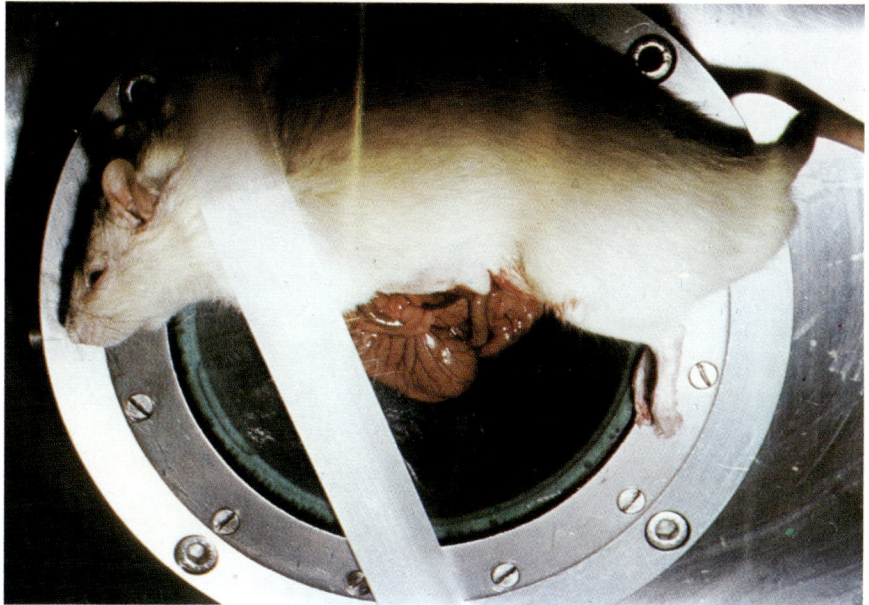

*Figure 16.* Experimental arrangement for the shock wave exposure of eventrated organs on the experimental table.

The series of following figures (17a-f) shows individual examples of this study however indicating that the shock wave exposure does not always result in disintegration of stones which spontaneously detach, mainly because the volume of the stone fragments was larger than the focus zone.

## 2.2.2 Rate and kinetic energy of stone fragments

In figures 18a and 18b the stone crumbling is shown in direct light. These studies show that the stone crumbling does not occur at the instant of entry of the shock wave but after a delay of several milliseconds. The rate of crumbling varies by small degrees with stones of varying chemical composition. However a dismantling of the structure was accomplished after 0.0025 second in every case.

Figures 19a-f present a cut of the high speed photography. (Motion photography of stone crumbling with a High-Cam high frequency camera. Frame exposure 1 microsecond).

1.4 microseconds after generating, the shock wave had traveled to the stone suspended in the focus. Only after 1-2 further microseconds is a dismantling of the structure of the concretion noticed. After 3 microseconds a pronounced

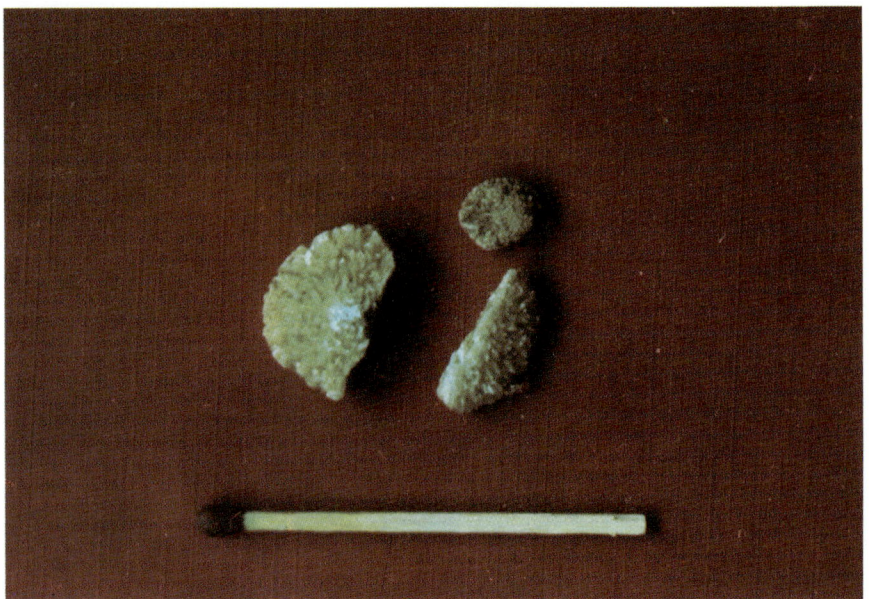

*a*

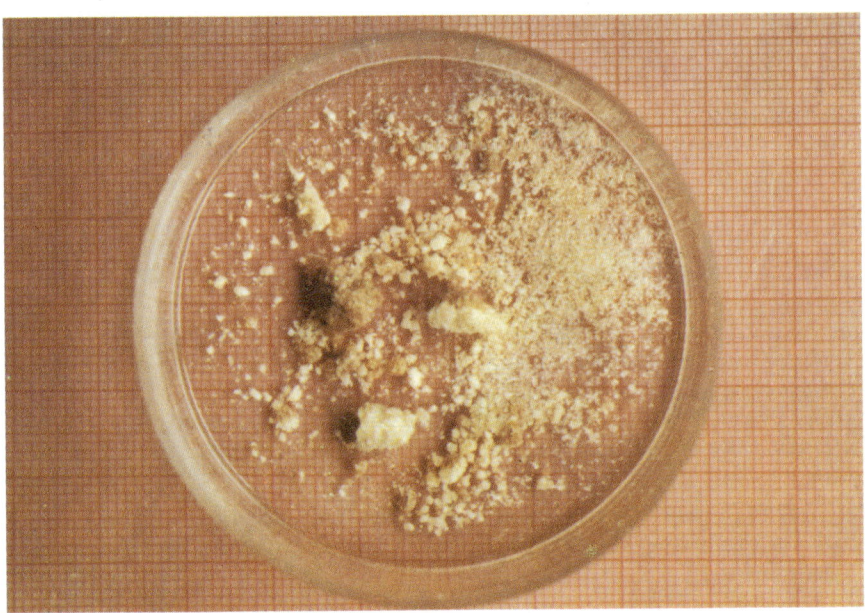

*b*
*Figure 17.* Calcium oxalate dihydrate stone before exposure (a) and after three shock wave exposures in the water bath (b). Voltage 27 kV, electrode separation 3.5 mm.

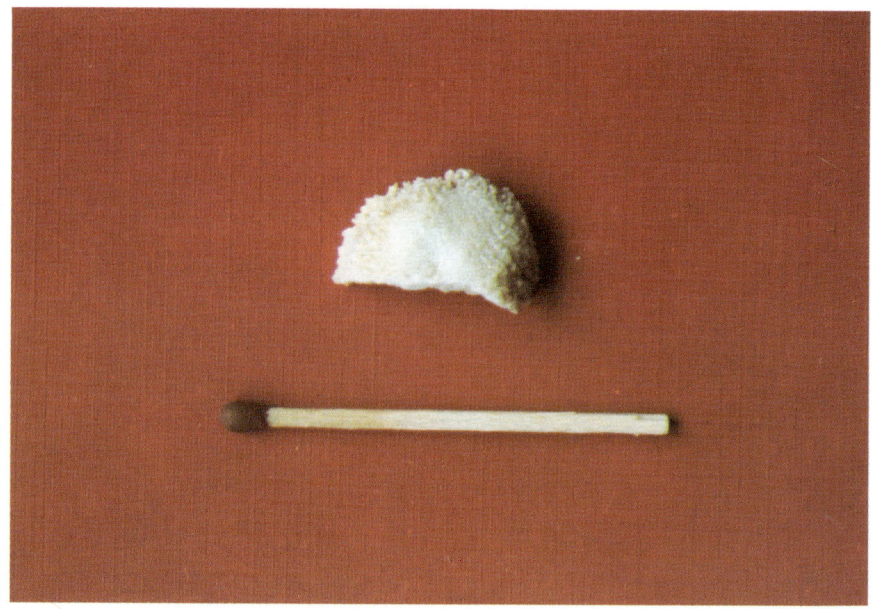

c

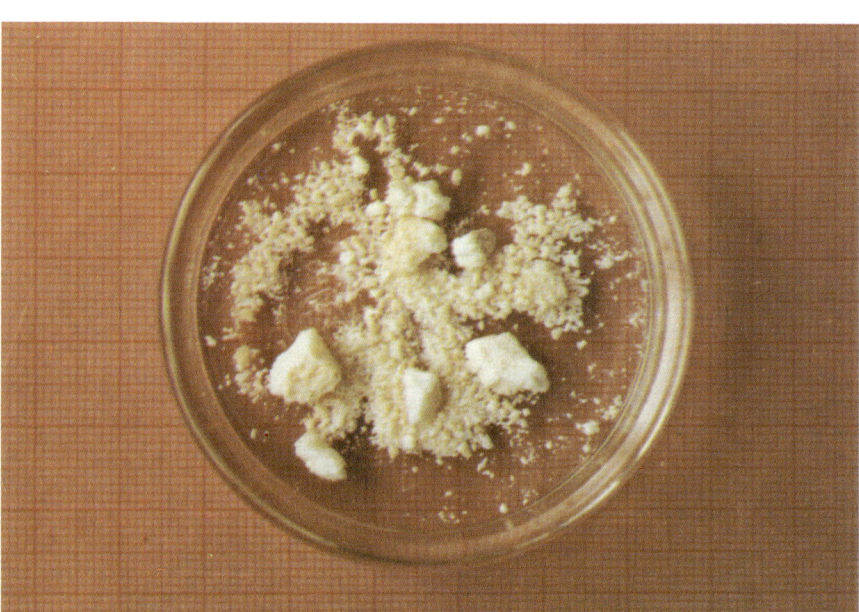

d

*Figure 17.* Magnesium ammomium phosphate stone before (c) and after three exposures (d). Voltage 27 kV, electrode separation 3.5 mm.

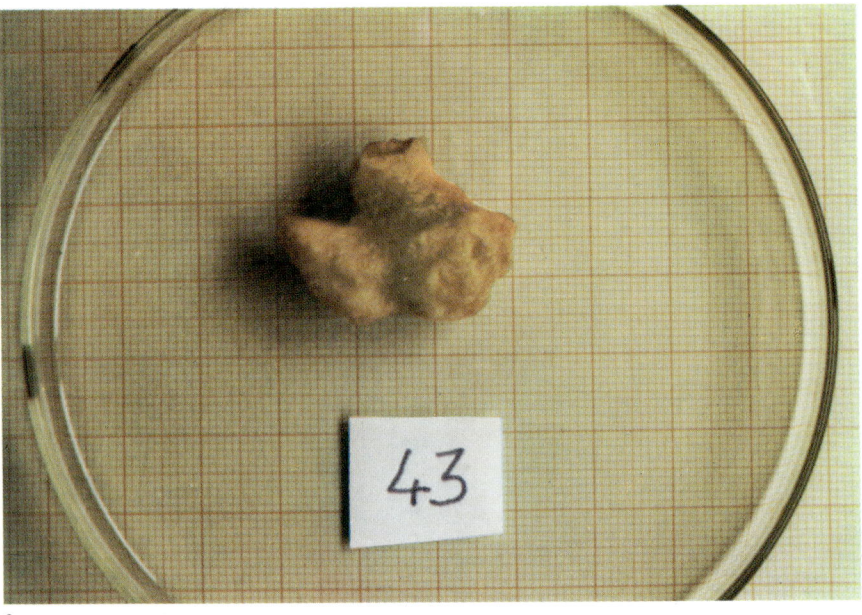

e

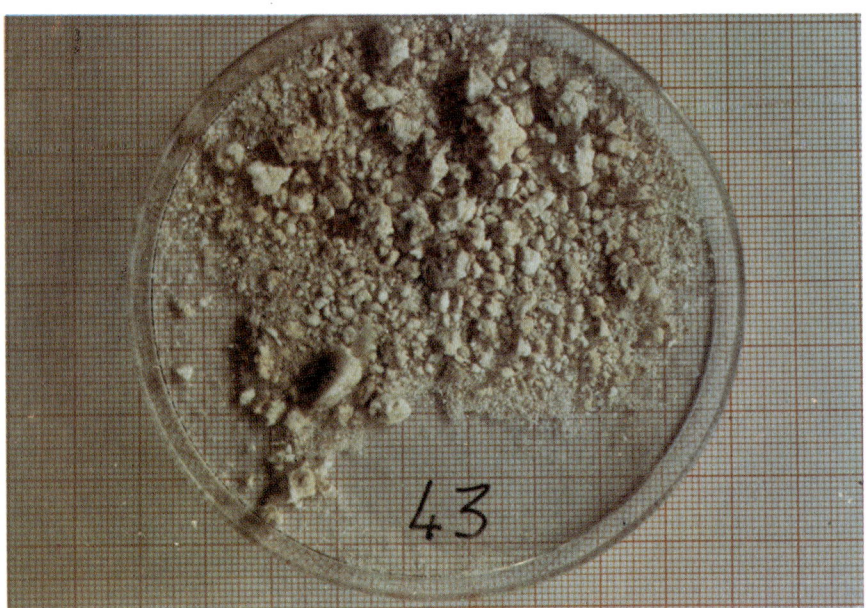

f

*Figure 17.* Tricalcium phosphate stone before (e) and after (f) two shock wave exposures.

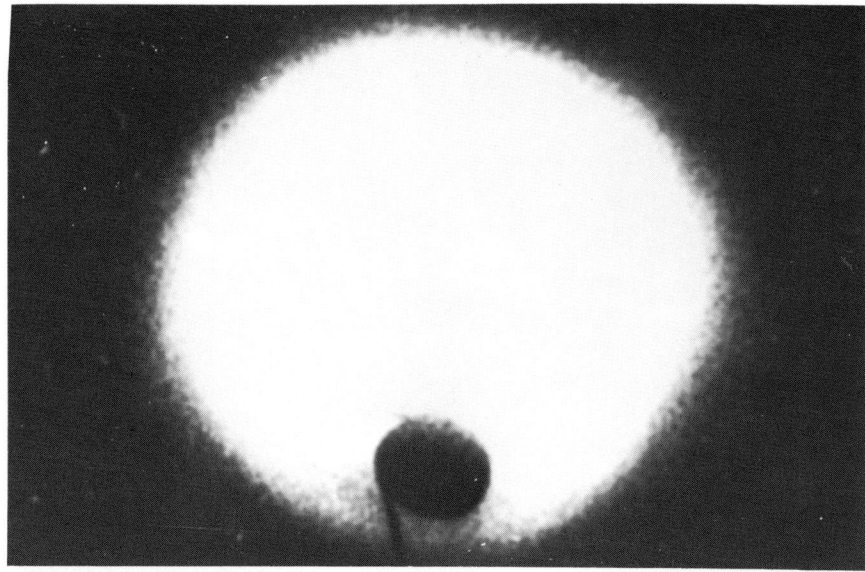

*a*

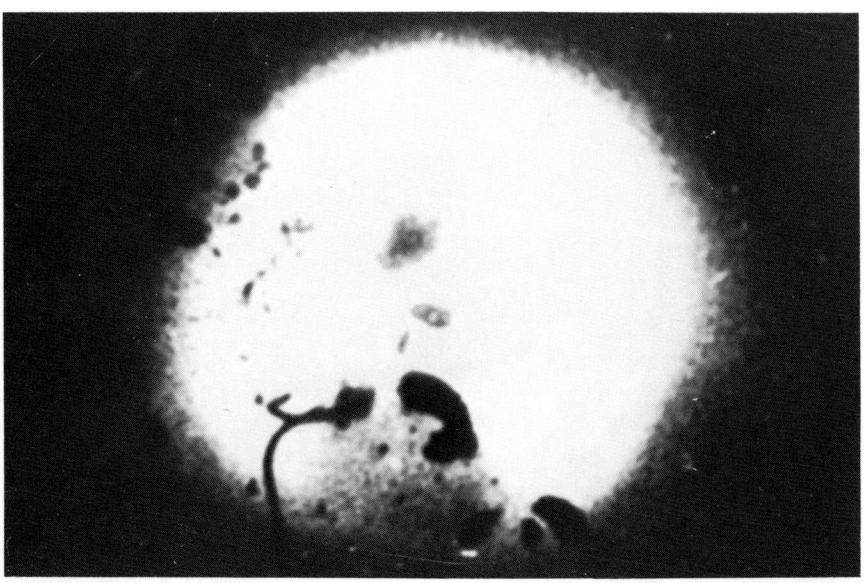

*b*

*Figure 18.* Photographic representation of stone crumbling in direct light. a) before exposure b) 0.0025 second after firing of the underwater spark gap. Type of stone: uric acid.

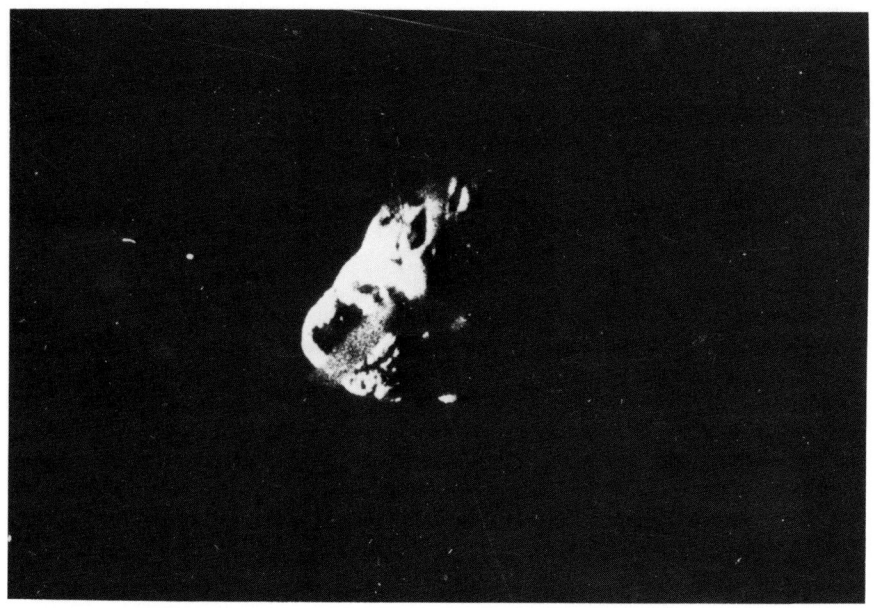

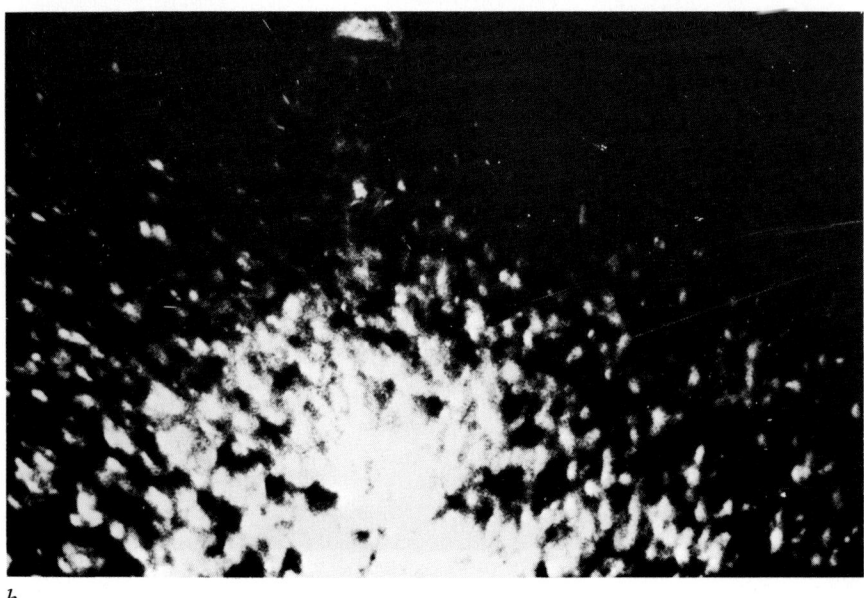

*Figure 19.* a) Stone before exposure (uric acid stone) b) 1 microsecond.

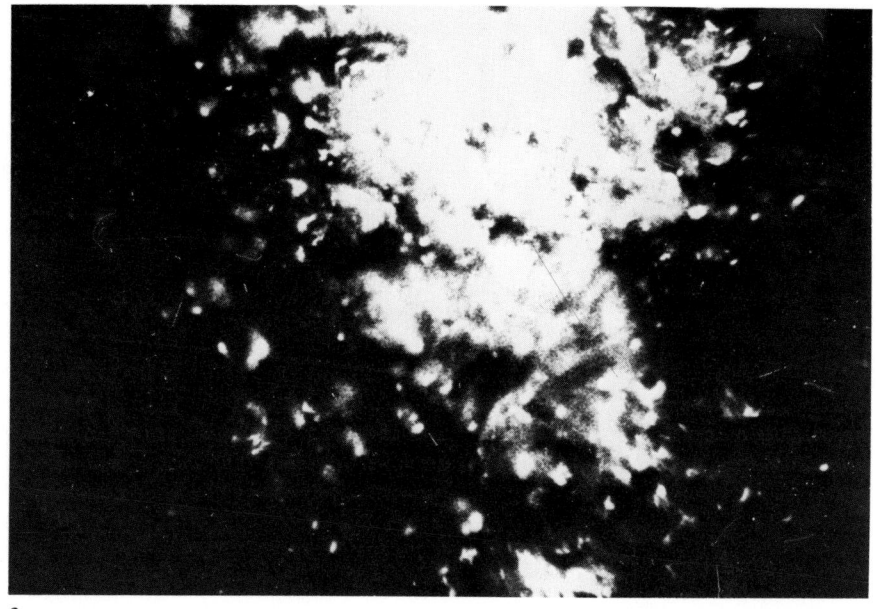

c

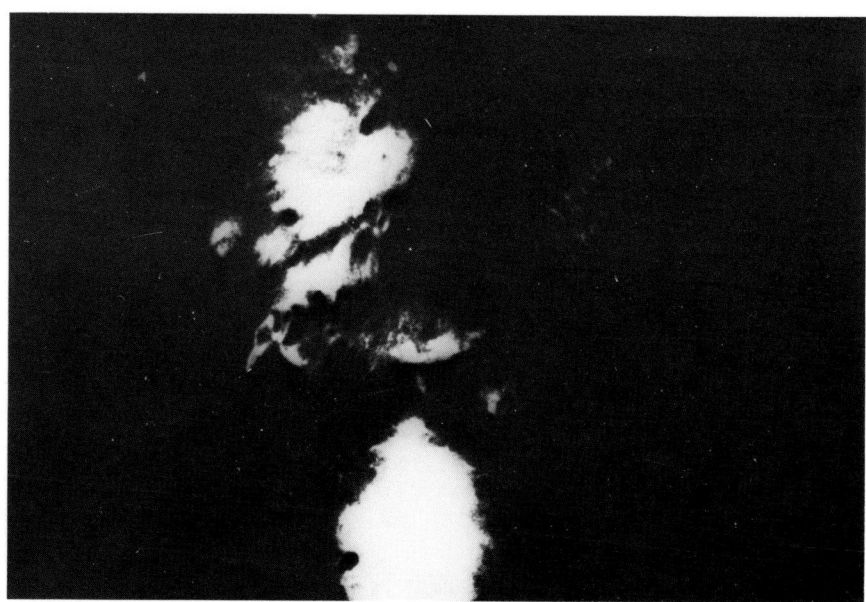

d

*Figure 19.* c) 2 microseconds d) 3 microseconds.

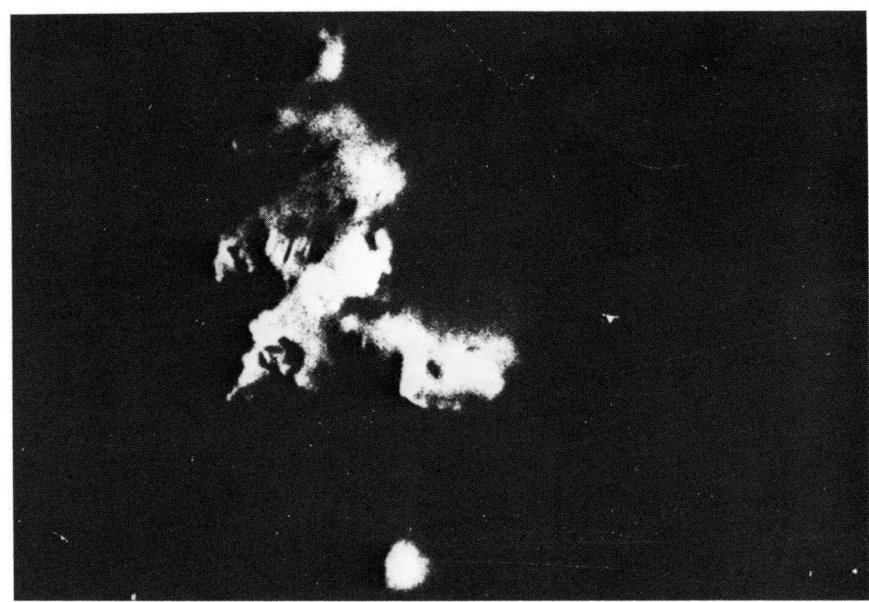

e

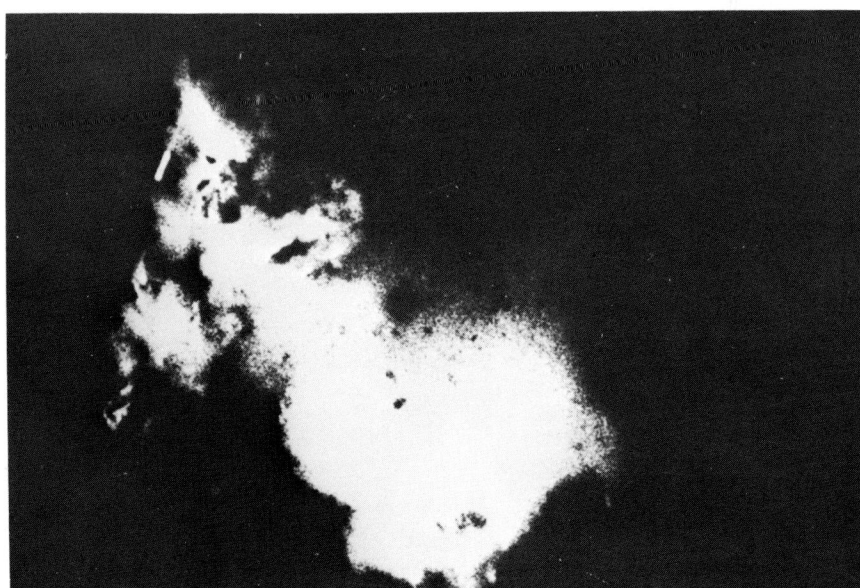

f

*Figure 19.* e) 4 microseconds f) 5 microseconds.

*Table III.* Rate (v) and kinetic energy (E) of stone fragments after shock wave exposure

| Figure | x (cm) | t ($10^{-3}$ sec) | $V_o$ (m/sec) | $E_{max.}$ ($10^{-3}$ J) |
|---|---|---|---|---|
| 19d | 1.07 | 2 | 5.4 | 2.3 |
| 19e | 1.25 | 3 | 4.2 | 1.4 |
| 19f | 1.75 | 4 | 4.3 | 1.5 |

dispersion of the individual fragments is seen which can have a speed of up to 5 m/sec. Based on the time sequence of the motion of the fragments away from the center, an average speed can be calculated and the kinetic energy of the dispersing fragments can also be found using the fragments' weights. Table III gives the values of the average speeds and kinetic energies of the fragments.

By these studies, fragments are found to have a maximum kinetic energy of $2 \times 10^{-3}$ Joule.

### 2.2.3 Evaluation of hemolysis

After several exposures of 10 ml of full blood, the plasmahemoglobin concentration was found to increase linearly in relation to the number of exposures up to 400 mg/100 ml after 4 exposures (figure 20).

It should be mentioned that a systematically demonstrable hemolysis could not be found in later animal studies, because the amount of the blood in the focus zone of the shock wave is too small in comparison to the whole volume for any

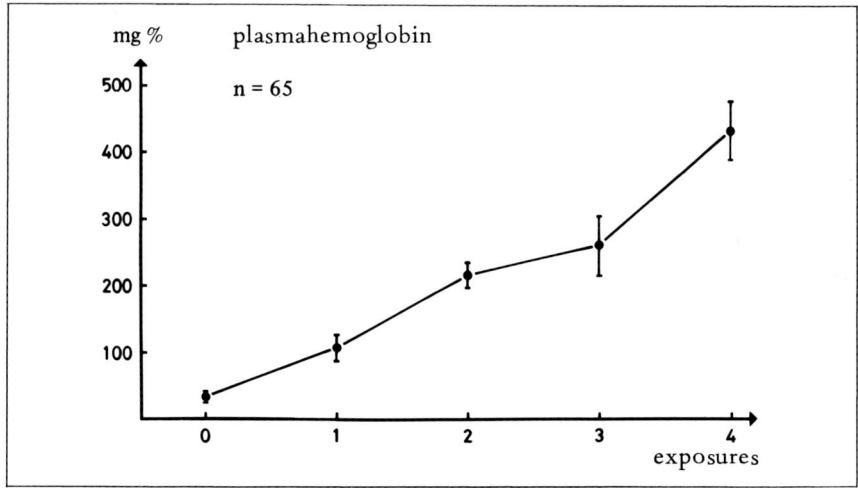

*Figure 20.* Behavior of plasma-hemoglobin concentration after repeated shock wave exposures.

effect to be noticed. Even after twenty exposures of the kidney area of the dog, no increase in free plasma-hemoglobin in the peripheral blood was measured.

### 2.2.4 Application of the shock waves to mixed lymphocyte cultures

No change in the count of lymphocytes was found between the counting done before and after exposure to the shock wave.

Neither was any change found in the stimulation capability of human lymphocytes which had been cultured after 2-5 exposures.

In table IV the test protocol of this series of experiments is given. No change in the stimulation rate could be observed after exposure either in the general mitogenetic stimulation with phythaemagglutinin (PHA) or in the mixed lymphocyte culture (MLC). Shock wave exposure has no influence on proliferative processes.

### 2.2.5 In vivo studies in rats (table V)

a) Thoracic exposure

With only a single exposure of the thoracic region a massive hemoptysis occured causing death of the research animals in every case. The histological studies of the collected lung tissues showed massive vascular and alveolar rupture. This effect can be avoided by covering the chest area with a 0.3 cm thick styrofoam sheet.

*Table IV.* Example of the stimulation study in the lymphocyte culture before and after shock wave exposure. Also given are the impulses per minute (cpm) and the quotient which is given from cpm (experimental) to cpm (untreated cells). Irradiated cells are marked with an x

| MLC 88 | Untreated cells | | Exposed cells | |
|---|---|---|---|---|
| | cpm | ratio | cpm | ratio |
| A+Ax | 2 708 | | 2 030 | |
| A+Bx | 87 849 | 32.4 | 57 325 | 28.2 |
| B+Bx | 2 515 | | 2 815 | |
| B+Ax | 102 274 | 40.6 | 142 317 | 50.2 |
| A control | 1 553 | | 1 250 | |
| A+PHA-P | 369 149 | 237 | 278 720 | 222 |
| B control | 1 506 | | 1 225 | |
| B+PHA-P | 382 314 | 253 | 367 775 | 300 |

*Table V.* Rat studies (+) in individual cases of petechial bleeding (+++) massive cell lesions

| Exposure 10 x | Clinical results | Pathological changes (24 hrs after experiment) | | Pathological changes (14 days after experiment) | |
|---|---|---|---|---|---|
| | | macro-scopic | micro-scopic | macro-scopic | micro-scopic |
| Thorax (n = 20) | massive hemoptysis | +++ | +++ | --- | --- |
| with a sheet of styrofoam (n = 20) | no result | ϕ | ϕ | ϕ | ϕ |
| Abdominal cavity (n = 20) | no result | ϕ | ϕ | ϕ | ϕ |
| Liver (n = 20) | no result | (+) | (+) | ϕ | ϕ |
| Colon | no result | (+) | (+) | ϕ | ϕ |

b) General exposure of the abdominal cavity

Even those animals exposed 10 times to the shock wave survived without any evidence of clinical damage. None of the entire group showed either macroscopic or microscopic pathological changes whether after 24 hours or 14 days.

c) Exposure of eventrated organs

*Large intestine:* After two exposures of the eventrated large intestine, isolated and widely disseminated petechial bleeding on the verge of the mesentery was observed. In no case were any massive bleeding or serous or intestinal wall lesions seen. All the animals of the long time group survived. With the histological preparation of the organs removed after 14 days there was no evidence of ill effects as a result of the trauma.

*Liver:* Here also, after two exposures, isolated petechial bleeding appeared. However in no case did these lesions lead to the death of the animal during the observation period of 14 days.

*Histology:* After 14 days no pathological changes were found in the morphological structure.

2.3  *Evaluation of the pretrial*

With the first shock wave device that was geared for the in vivo and in vitro studies of small animals it was proven that:

1. urinary stones with different chemical compositions could be reproducibly destroyed contact-free with the application of shock waves;
2. in clinical application there was no traumatizing of biological tissues by the shock wave exposure whether in vivo or in vitro.

# 3. Studies for experimental in vivo stone destruction – Development of an apparatus for experimental in vivo stone destruction

After the previously described biological and medical pretrials, problems in conducting further experimental procedures appeared. With the goal in mind of clinical application, the solution was an adequate experimental arrangement. The main requirements in order to further develop these methods for clinical usage are, as follows.

1. Integration of a positioning device for the exact location of the kidney stone and lining up the concretion in the focal region.
2. Development of a stone model for animal experiments which simulates human stone disease.
3. Development of a prototype for larger animal studies by which in vivo kidney stone destruction will be possible.

## 3.1 Methods

### 3.1.1 Integration of an ultrasonic location system

Three ultrasonic transducers were placed in the ellipsoid through a hole bored in the side, whose axes intersect in the objective focal region of the shock waves. The oscillating axes of the transducers are placed symmetrically on either side of the major axis of the semi-ellipsoid at an angle of 30° (figure 21).

The individual ultrasonic transducer can act as either a transmitter or a receiver or it can be used in a single function mode. In the first case, ultrasonic echoes were recorded, which are known from ultrasonic diagnostics as A-images. Through the separation of the transmitter and the receiver in this procedure a modified A-image will be created. The ultrasonic impulse is sent by one transducer and reflected echoes having an angle of 30° are received at the second ultrasonic transducer.

A frequency of 2.25 MHz was selected for the ultrasonic transducer which has a diameter of 20 mm. This gives a close range of 13.5 cm. With a distance of 16 cm from the objective focus to the ultrasonic transducer surface, the objective focal point lies at the beginning of the wide range. The diameter of the "sound lobe" is 23 mm in the objective focus. Model stones (diameter = 5-15mm) of various sizes were placed in a homogeneous medium (water) at the focal point and the amplitude of the reflected echoes was determined. This was done in order to answer the question of what the received echo intensity would be and the dispersing properties of the device would be.

In a further study, these model stones were placed under a layer of tissue in order to determine what echoes would be produced by tissue transmission.

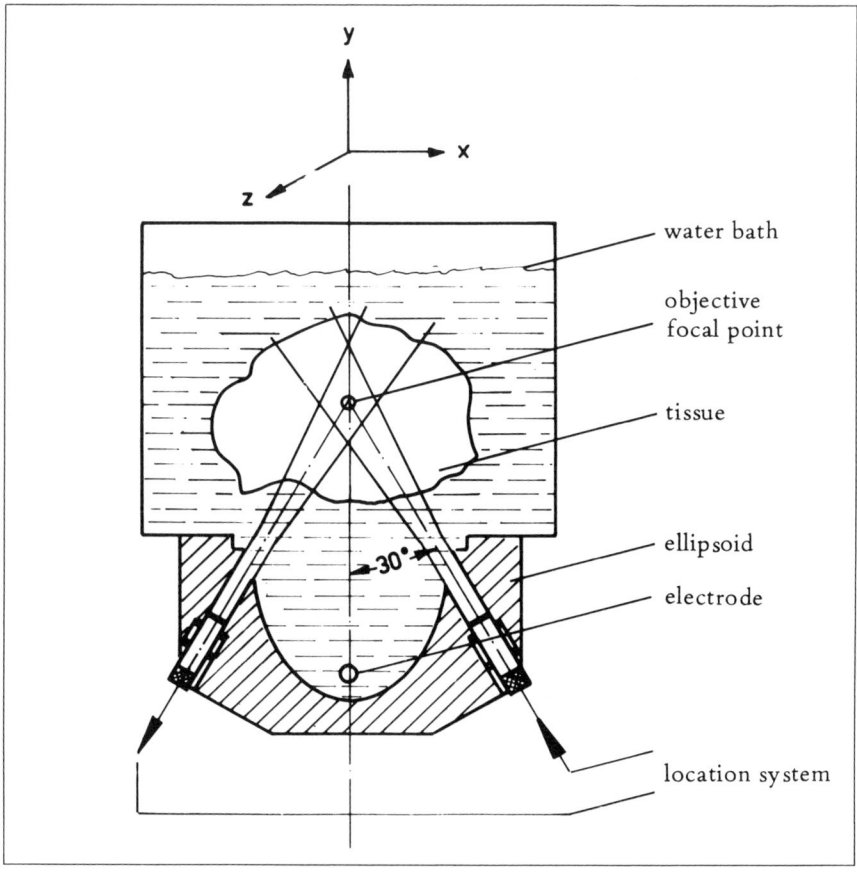

*Figure 21.* Schematic representation of the ultrasonic transducers in the semi-ellipsoid.

### 3.1.2 Integration of an ultrasonic B-scanner

The A-image yields only information concerning the studied object along the symmetry axis of the ultrasonic transducer. Points of light are allocated to the amplitudes of the A-image and displayed on a screen so that the characteristic spectrum of an impulse echogram along the axis of symmetry is created. Through displacement or swinging of the ultrasonic transducer, it is possible to construct a two dimensional image out of these light points. This procedure is known as B-imaging.

For integration of a B-scanner, an apparatus was used that has a small coupling surface. We used an ultrasonic imaging system from the firm *Picker*-Roentgen.

The transducer was fastened in a rubber collar and brought through an opening

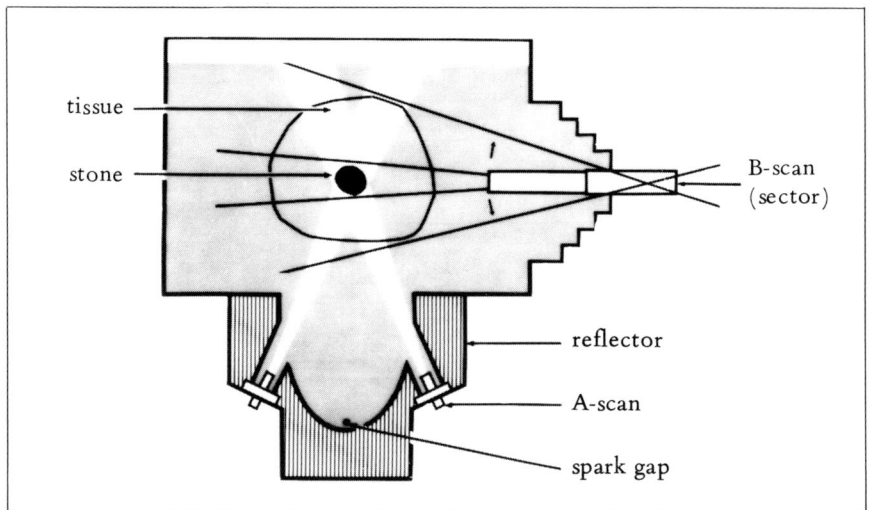

*Figure 22.* Schematic representation of the integration of a B-scan ultrasonic location system in the experimental apparatus.

in the side of the water bath (figure 22). Through this holder the necessary movements of the transducer were not influenced. The real-time sections received were transverse sections of the experimental animal.

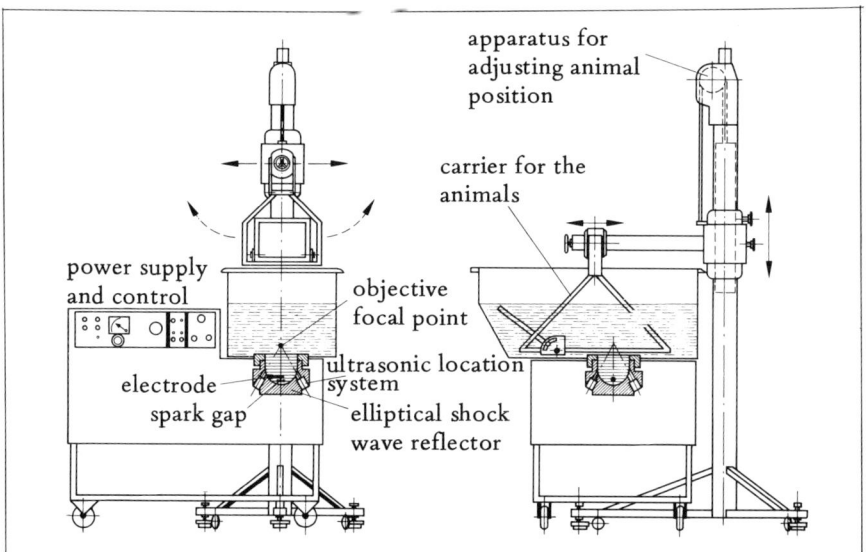

*Figure 23.* Shock wave generator model 1. Schematic representation.

## 3.1.3 Experimental apparatus

Figure 23 shows the schematic representation of the first prototype for large animal studies.

Besides minor technical changes in the wiring (for example, a reduction of the total inductance of the switching circuit of up to 155 nH), the structural changes were mainly an enlargement of the trial chamber (40-50x120 cm) and the integration of a suspension and an adjustment device, with which the research animals could be positioned over the focal region.

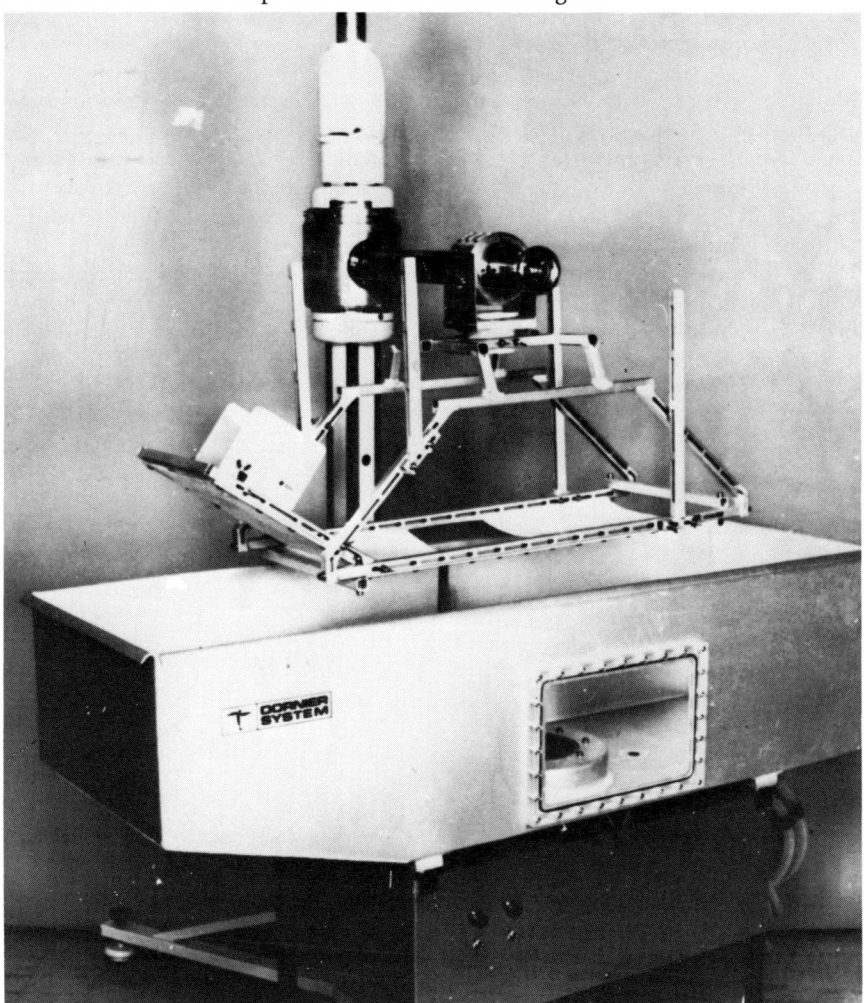

*Figure 24.* Photographic representation of the experimental container with the attached underwater spark generator and device for positioning the research animals.

The device has two independent components: the shock wave generator with the experimental compartment and the flanged semi-ellipsoid with the underwater spark generator and with a freely moving device for positioning the research animals (figure 24).
Based on the mobility of the coupling links, which are indicated in the picture by arrows, it is possible to position the research animal anywhere desired over the ellipsoid. The adjustment can be made within a few millimeters by positioning gears.

*3.1.4 Experimental stone model*

Mongrels with a weight of 15-20 kg were anesthetized with pentobarbital (25 mg/kg-BW), and a tracheal tube was introduced. Under sterile conditions, a pararectal laparotomy was performed, and the right ureter was located and ligatured approximately 1 cm above the entrance to the bladder. Afterwards the wound was closed layer by layer and the animal was placed under intensive antibiotic and infusion therapy during a postoperative period.
Under the same anesthetic, the animals were again laparotomized 8 days later with a median incision, and the right kidney cavity was prepared. A very pronouncedly dilated kidney cavity was revealed, in which were implanted by a longitudinal pyelotomy human kidney stones with a diameter of 1-1.5 cm.

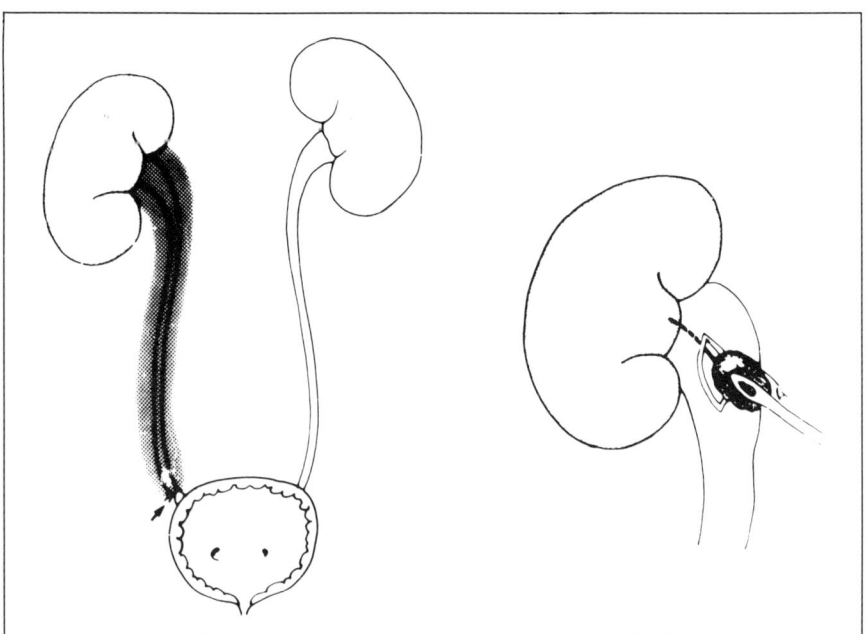

*Figure 25.* Experimental procedure for the implantation of human kidney stones in the renal pelvic calyx system of the dog.

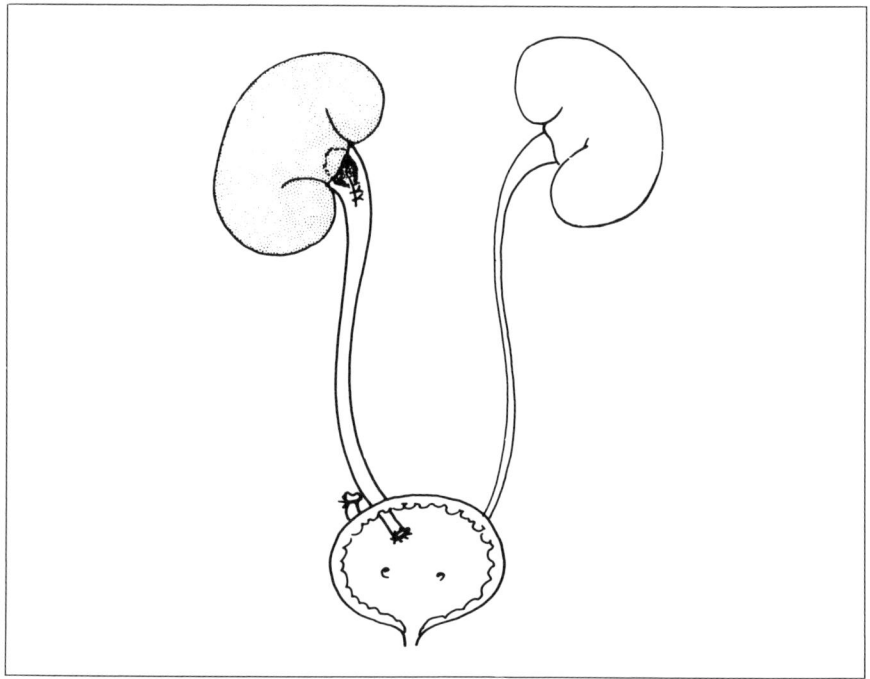

*Figure 26.* Situation after the stone implantation and ureteroneocystostomy.

Because postoperative control was accomplished by X-ray, stones which gave X-ray images were employed (oxalate stones). The pyelon and retroperitoneal cavity were closed with individual sutures. After the sutures were put in, the ligature on the ureter was cut and the ureter was reimplanted in the bladder without antireflux plastic (figure 26). The X-ray control was conducted postoperatively at one week intervals.

### 3.1.5 Animal studies

With this apparatus 45 studies of 35 kidney stone carrying and 10 untreated animals were done.
The anesthetized animal was placed on its side in the suspension device and positioned by the adjusting mechanisms at the focal point region of the ellipsoid. By placing the ultrasonic transducers and with the vertical movement of the B-scan oscillator the location was adjusted until the stone echo fell in the focal region. After this, the animals received from one to ten shock wave exposures. In cases where there was no clear echo of the implanted concretion, a more general exposure of the right kidney was performed. After the conclusion of

the experiment, X-ray examination was conduced for the evaluation of the effect of the exposure and was repeated on a weekly basis to evaluate the breakdown of the individual pieces.

An evaluation of the possible organic damage caused by shock waves in animals with implanted kidney stones was made difficult by secondary effects in the nature of inspecific inflammation in stone kidneys.

To verify the results found in small animals in dog models 10 non-stone carrying animals were exposed in the kidney area to 10 shock wave treatments. 48 hours after the studies a section was conducted, and after macroscopic evaluation of the tissue samples of the kidney, liver, spleen, pancreas, duodenum, colon, lung, rib, and spinal cord, histologic studies were performed.

## 3.2 Results

### 3.2.1 Stone implantation

65 dogs were operated on using the specified stone implantation method. With the exception of two animals, which after 8 days still did not demonstrate sufficient blockage of the kidney cavity system, the implantation of 1-2 cm human oxalate stones was performed without complications in all cases.

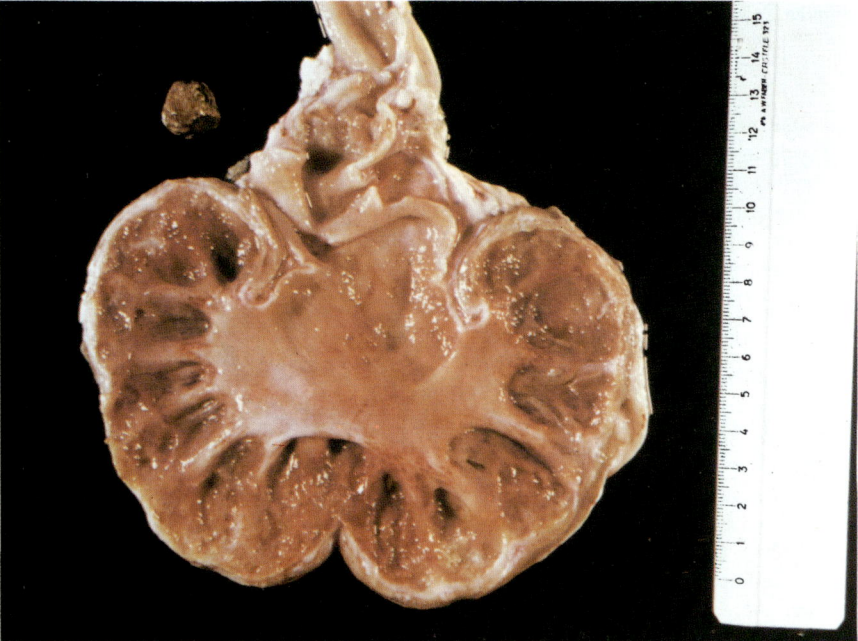

*Figure 27.* Pyonephrosis due to stone blockage after implantation.

4 animals died from urosepsis proceeding from the stone kidney. Sectioning revealed a sack-like pyonephrosis because the out flow had been completely blocked by the stone having entered the ureter (figure 27). Figure 28 is one of a series of X-rays taken postoperatively, in this case after seven days; the concretion may be seen as the shadow in the right kidney area.

Accordingly, the urogram shows, 20 minutes after injection of the dye, the concretion in the kidney cavity with a slightly dilated pelvis.

Figures 30a and b give another example of a stone successfully implanted in the kidney cavity, where it led to no changes of the pelvis of the kidney since it was discharged in time.

Approximately 70 % of the surgeries which were conducted led, three weeks after implantation, to a complete regression of the urinary blockage. In 25 % of the animals there was a slight urinary blockage of the kidney either from a delaying of drainage from the implanted stone or from a restricturing in the area of the implantation.

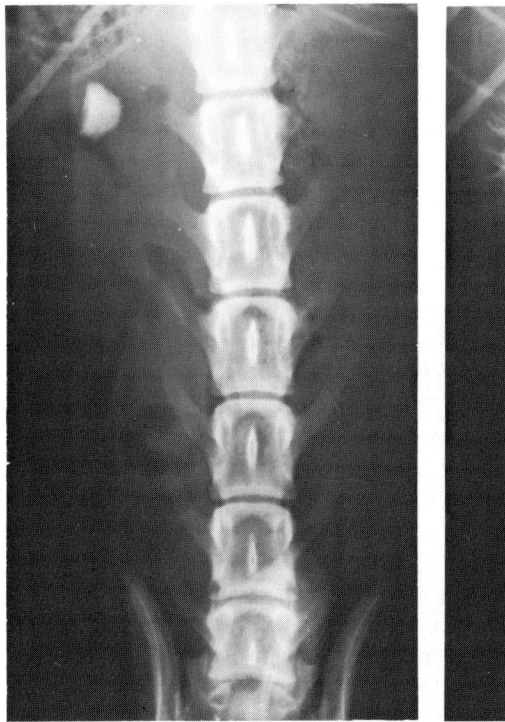
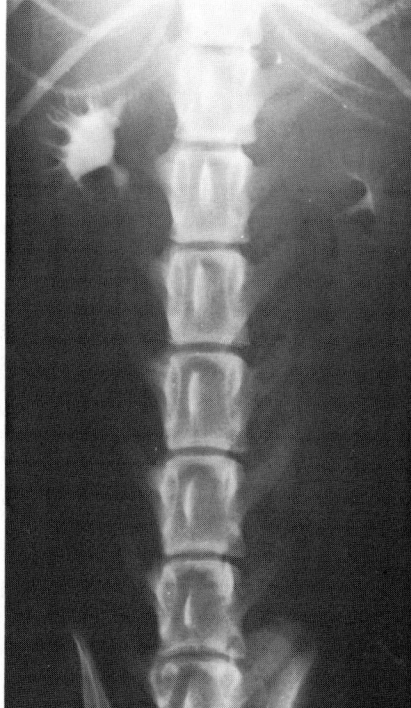

*Figure 28.* Radiogram on the seventh day after implantation of a human calcium oxalate stone.

*Figure 29.* Urogram: Photograph 20 minutes after the dye injection. Discharge in time with slight blockage of the kidney cavity system.

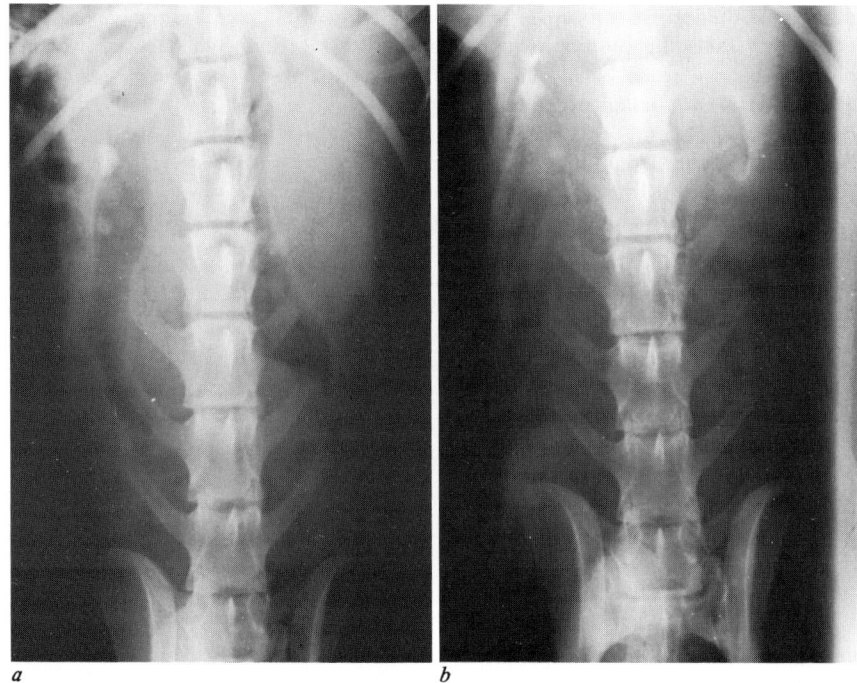

*Figure 30.* a) X-ray plate 7 days after the kidney stone implantation on the right. b) Urogram after stone implantation with dye discharge on time and not dilated collecting system.

Figure 31 shows a section prepared four weeks after stone implantation. The longitudinally sectioned kidney with the calcium oxalate stone lying in the kidney cavity shows no changes in the renal pelvis.

*3.2.2 Integration of the ultrasonic location system*

a) A-scanner

The influence of the stone size on the amplitude of the echo signal is given in figure 32. The echo intensity is reduced tenfold for every twofold reduction in the size of the kidney stone. This result is still reproducible even when the transmitter and receiver are switched among the three integrated transducers. A useful echo can be obtained down to a stone size of r = 5 mm.

b) Modified A-scanner

By adding a tissue layer between the ultrasonic transducer and the concretion, the echoes that result as the signal enters and leaves the tissue are superimposed

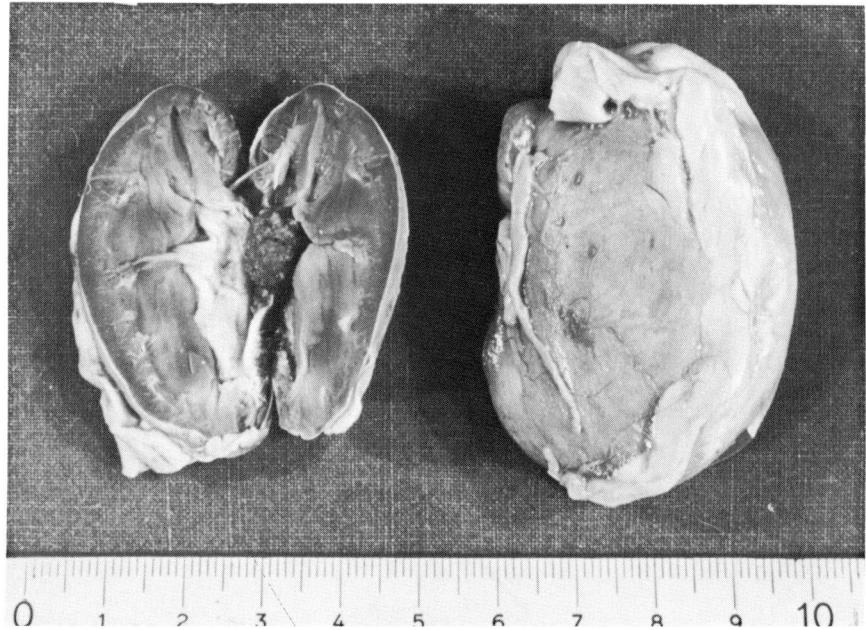

*Figure 31.* A prepared section of a dog kidney four weeks after implantation of a human kidney stone.

on the echo signal actually received from the stone (one ultrasonic transducer is a synchronized transmitter and receiver). By separating the transmitter from the receiver these interfering signals can be suppressed to an extent.

In addition there were multiple reflections between the study animal and the transducer, which as interfering artifacts made the analysis of the stone echoes more difficult. Through a flexible arrangement of these transducers in a telescope system these reflections could be suppressed by changing the distance the sound travels between the animal and the transducer.

*In vitro location*

In in vitro studies it was possible in each case to locate the stone through the tissue layer, to position it in the focus zone and consequently destroy it by means of the shock wave exposures (figure 33). But it was not possible in these studies to obtain sufficiently effective control of the shock wave impact by means of an ultrasound image.

*In vivo location*

With stones that were implanted in the kidney cavity, the clearly interpretable ultrasonic signal was the exception. Figure 34 shows the ultrasonic echogram

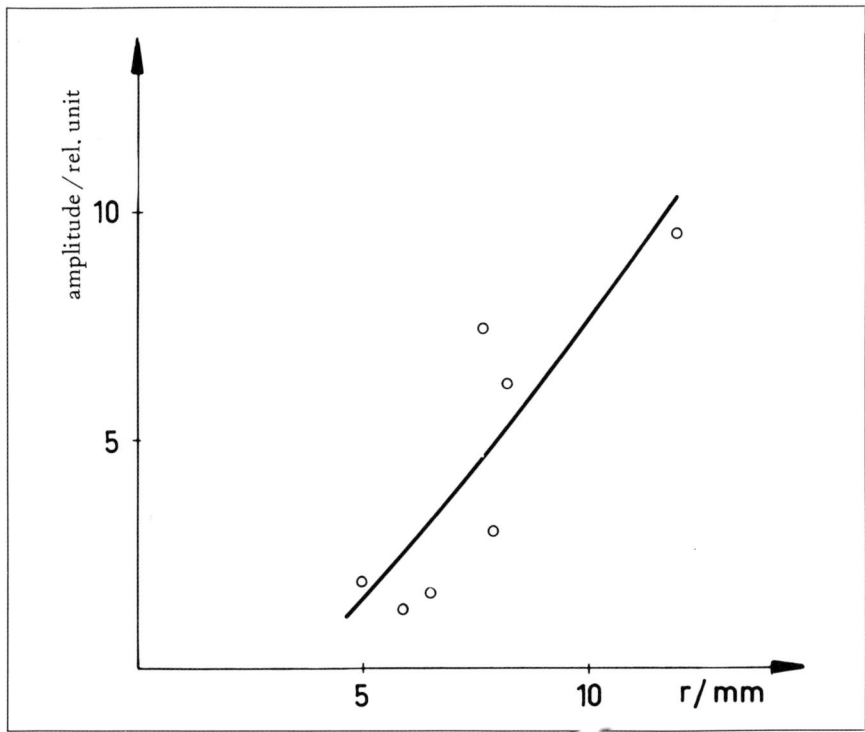

*Figure 32.* Amplitude of the ultrasonic signal with changing stone size.

of a stone which has spontaneously displaced into the ureter after implantation. Because the concretion was located only a few centimeters under the surface of the skin, there was no creation of interfering echos, and a sufficient peak co-ordinating signal at the stone was not hindered. Such a stone localization was the exception, and the end result of these studies determined that a localization using the A-scan procedure which gives results sufficiently reproducible for clinical use was not possible.

c) B-scanner

*In vitro studies*

Human kidney stones, placed in swine kidneys in the model study, were localized using both the A-scan and the B-scan procedure. The 14 and 8 mm size stones produced a clear, recognizable echo and the echo-free cast shadow (sound cancellation behind the stone, fig. 35) typical for such a structure.

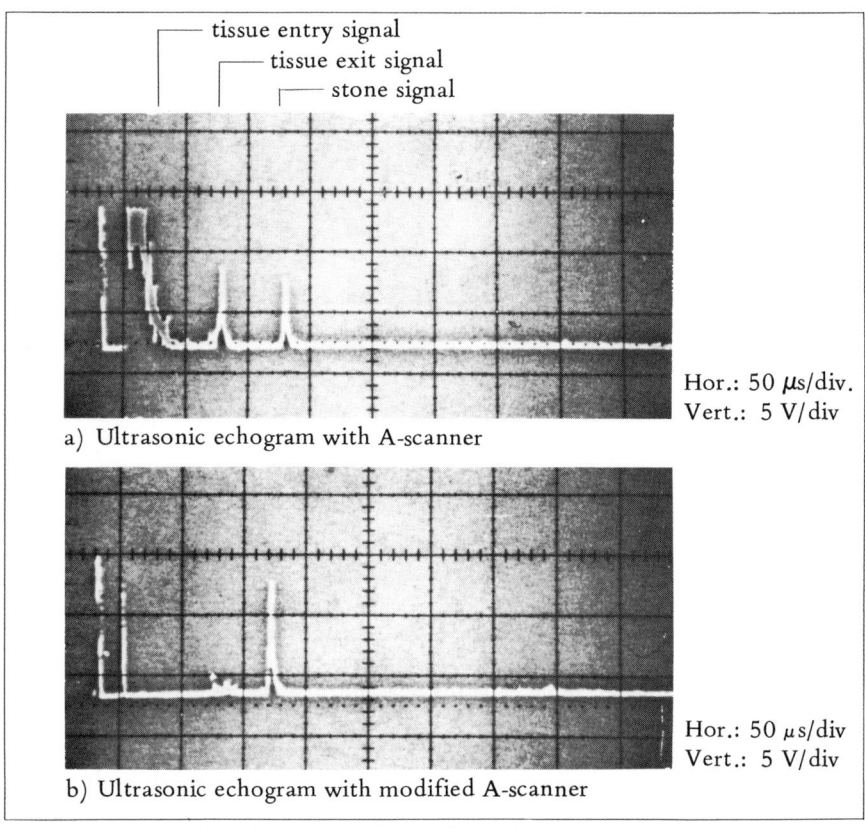

Figure 33. Stone location in vitro in a swine kidney.

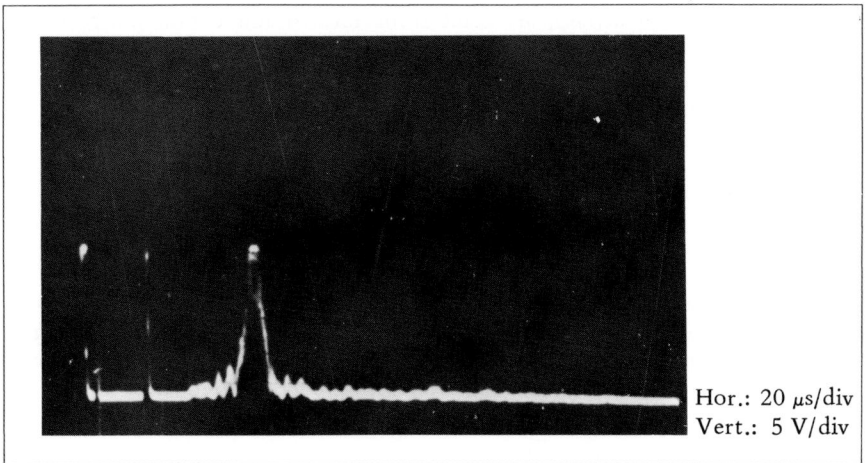

Figure 34. Ultrasonic echogram of a ureter stone with modified A-scanner.

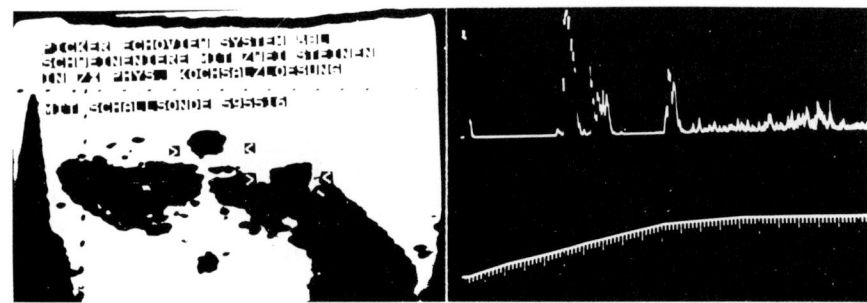

*Figure 35.* Sonogram with presentation of the kidney stone in vitro studies. Left: B-scan signal, right: A-scan signal.

*In vivo studies*

The selected distance of the ultrasonic transducer for the in vivo studies is 10 cm. This brought about a useful penetration of 10 cm, because the echoes returning from deeply situated body tissues coincided with repeating echoes, for example those from the interface of the water and skin, and rendered the signals unanalyzable. Figures 36a and b show sonograms from dogs after kidney stone implantation.
In both figures a well-defined outline of the kidney and a sharply defined pelvis can be recognized. Stone location still could not be achieved, however, because the shadow zone necessary for identification was superimposed by the repeating signals.
By using the B-scan procedure the advantage exists that the kidney outline and the pelvis can be identified, an exact stone localization within the realm of millimeters is not possible as is needed for clinical application. Artefacts arising from the repeating echoes interfere with the cast shadow arising from the stone and make the diagnosis impossible.

### 3.2.3 In vivo studies of stone destruction

a) Shock wave exposure of non-stone bearing animals

With the macroscopic evaluation, there were no changes of the exposed kidney and surrounding structures. In a few cases slight bleeding in the area of the right lower lung lobe was observed. But in no case did a hemothorax arise. (These studies, which have just been mentioned, were conducted with a general screen exposure so that exposure of the lung was unavoidable.)

With the histological study of the kidney and the surrounding organs there were no pathological results.

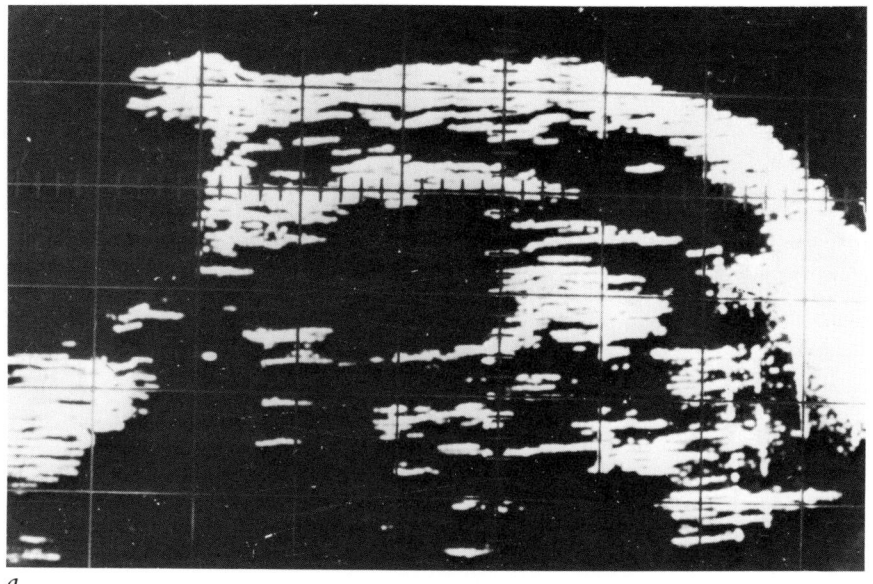

a

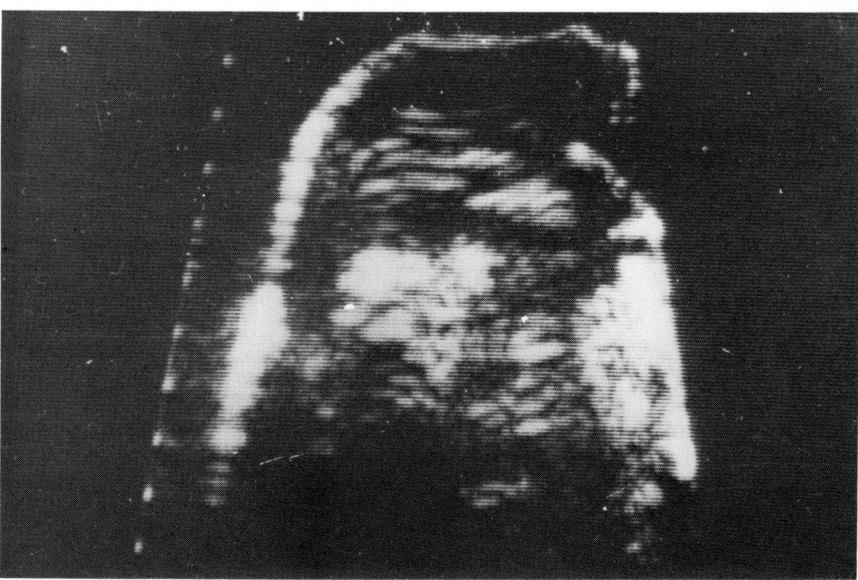

b

*Figure 36.* Transverse sonogram of the right kidney section of a dog after stone implantation. a) bistable screen indicator. b) half-tone image.

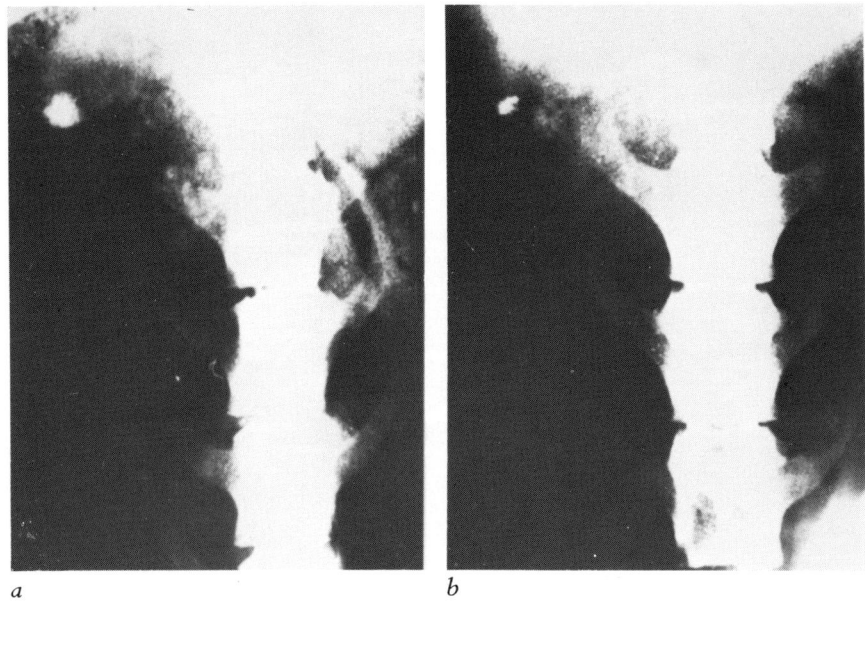

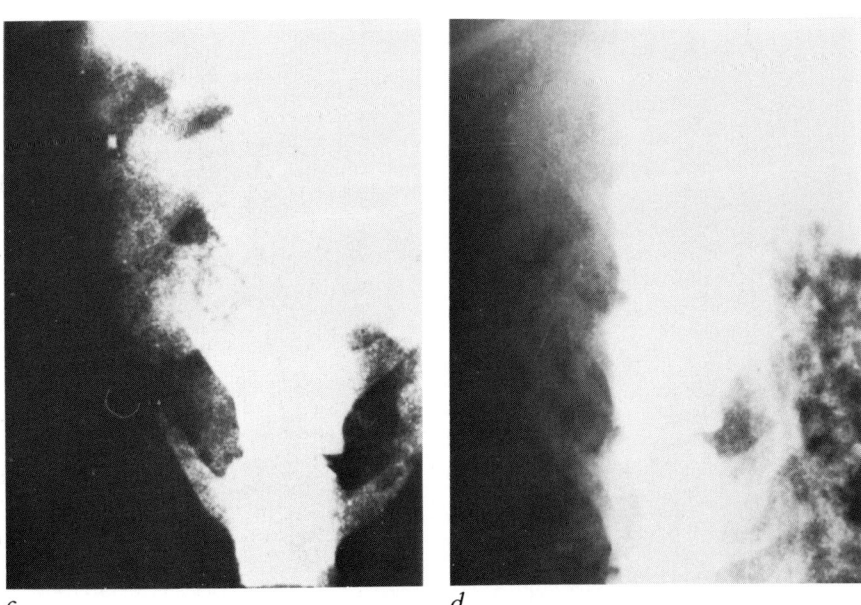

*Figure 37.* 4 week monitor photographs after shock wave exposure of an implanted calcium oxalate stone. a) before the study. b) - d) 4 weeks after the study.

In two study animals, because of their size, the area contralateral to the exposure side was not immersed in water. In these cases the contralateral side did show some discrete, petechial bleeding subcutaneously. This did not happen to any animal which was completely submerged.

b) In vivo stone destruction

As has already been described, there was a reliable localization of the implanted kidney stone by means of the ultrasonic system which was employed only in a few cases. In 80 % there was an unfocused area of bombardment above the stone bearing kidney.

Nevertheless it was possible in all cases to achieve a crumbling of the stone structure. As can be seen in the following figures the individual pieces of the concretions varied greatly. It was possible in 4 animals even through a general exposure to disintegrate the stone to such an extent that it was spontaneously discharged within 14 days (figure 37).

Figure 38 shows an example of the exposure of a spontaneously discharged oxalate stone in the ureter, where an ultrasonic location was possible.

After localizing, the stone was exposed twice with the result that it separated into two clearly identifiable pieces. Three further exposures shock waves led to a further disintegration of the concretion, so that a spontaneous discharge

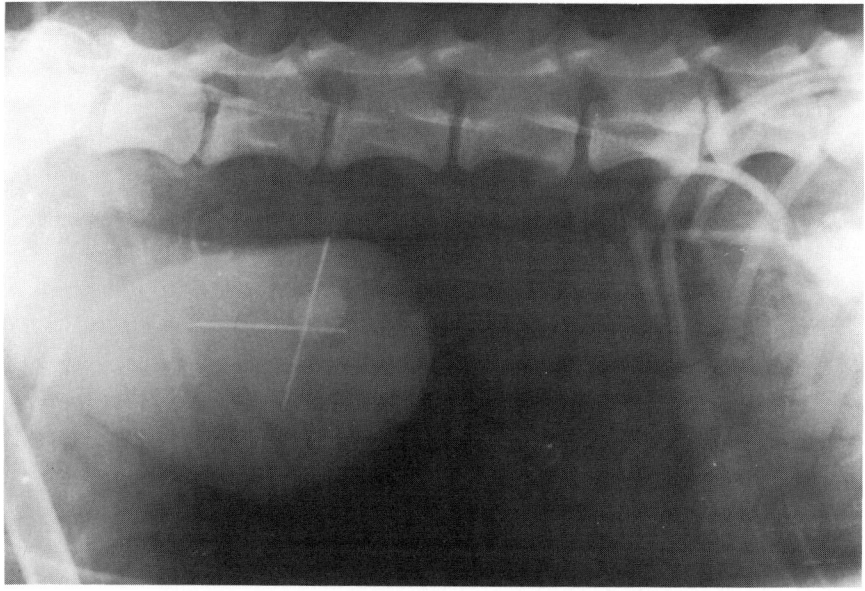

*Figure 38.* Photograph of a spontaneously discharged calcium oxalate stone in the ureter before the study.

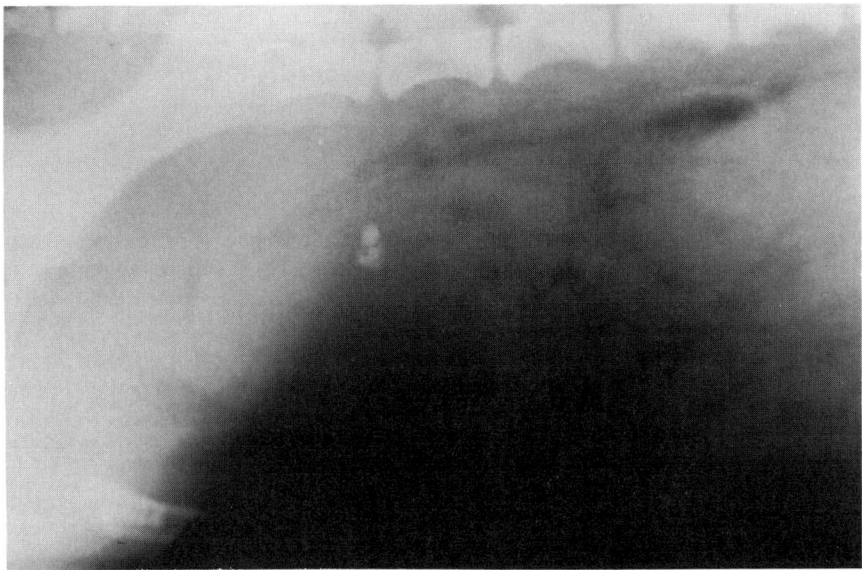

a

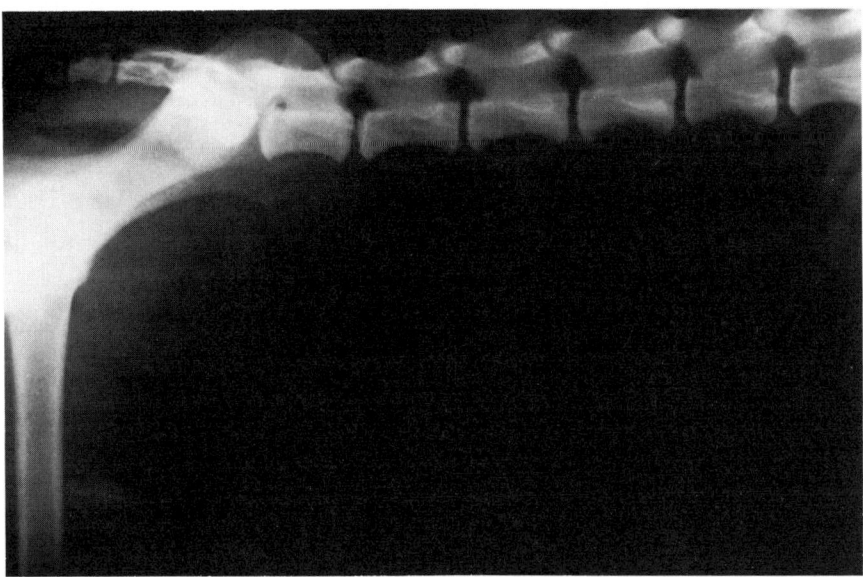

b

*Figure 39.* a) Photograph after 2 exposures to shock waves. The fragments of the stone may be noticed in the ureter and in the urethra. b) Photograph two weeks after another shock wave exposure, no fragments can be seen in the X-ray.

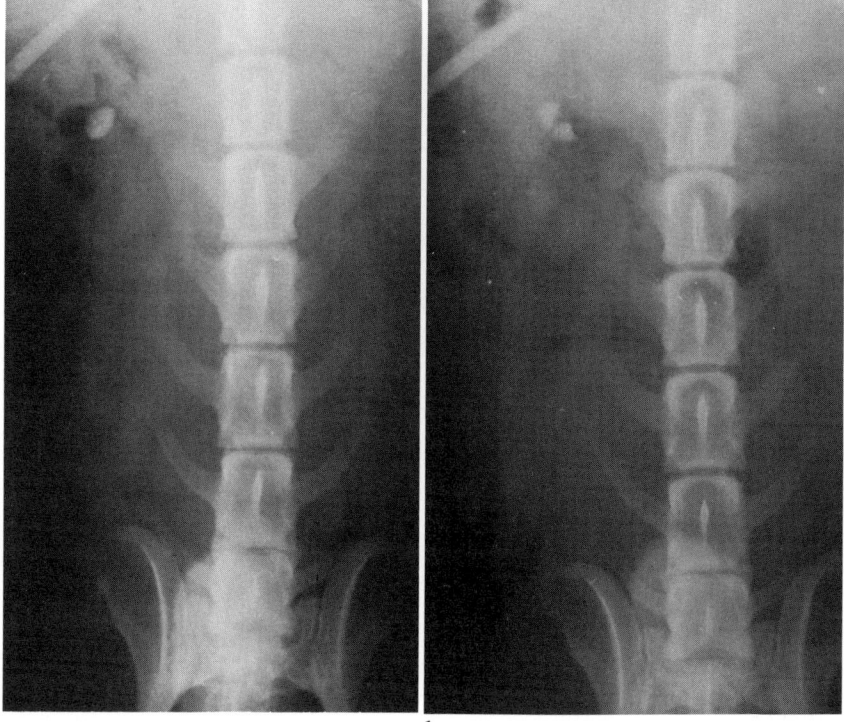

*a*            *b*

*Figure 40.* X-ray before (a) and after (b) 10 shock wave exposures (general exposure).

through the ureter was possible. In figure 39a the individual pieces can be recognized in the urethra while two even smaller fragments can be located in the ureter. Figure 39b shows that after 14 more days no more stones may be seen.

Successful stone destruction and consequent stone discharge were observed only in isolated cases in this study series. In the other 90 % it was possible to destroy the stones, but such large individual concretions remained that spontaneous discharge was not possible (figures 40a and b).

If another shock wave exposure was conducted on these animals, the possibility of a focused exposure was much less because now the size of the concretions was much smaller. There was a further disintegration of the concretion fragments with a new application of the shock waves. But this led to a complete alleviation of the stones in only four examples.

The histological studies, a few animals being observed for up to a year, showed no pathological modification which could be attributed to the shock wave application.

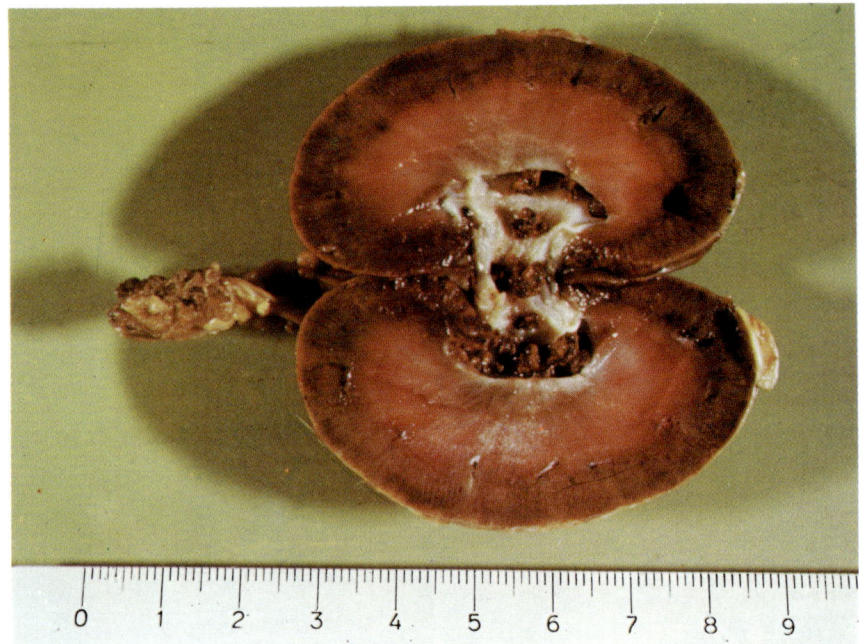

*Figure 41.* Prepared section of a stone bearing dog kidney immediately after shock wave exposure.

Figure 41 shows a prepared section immediately after shock wave exposure in which the small individual pieces from the concretion are seen. Whether with macroscopic or microscopic examination, no lesion was found immediately after exposure in the surrounding urothelium.

3.3  *Evaluation of the first large animal studies*

1. It is possible to disintegrate in vivo urinary concretions without direct contact with the energy source by transmitting high energy shock waves.
2. Neither by destroying the stone nor by direct contact with the shocks does traumatization to the kidney and surrounding tissues result.
3. But not in each case is it possible to obtain a disintegration of the concretions into dischargeable pieces by exposures with pressure amplitudes up to 2-3 kbar.
4. Through the integration of an ultrasonic location system reproducible stone location is not possible. With an integrated B-scan procedure it is possible to see the outline of the kidney and the pelvis, but clear stone identification is not possible.

# 4. Preclinical shock wave applicator

The results described in part three determined the need for technical changes on the apparatus, specifically, the next two points.

1. An improvement of stone location. Our use of the available technology of ultrasound did not permit the precise location of stones. Therefore an X-ray system coupled to the shock wave device was studied to see if a more reliable concretion location could be reached.
2. The shock wave application in the selected form led to a stone crumbling but it was not always possible to reach pieces of the size that are spontaneously discharged. Tests needed to be conducted to obtain a diminishing of the concretion size by changing the pressure amplitude.

Only after these problems could be solved it was possible to envisage clinical application.

## 4.1 Methods

### 4.1.1 Prestudies of X-ray location

Before deciding to integrate an extremely expensive device for X-ray location into the shock wave device, studies were conducted on the influence of the intervening water on the resolution capacity of the X-ray device and the appearance of the implanted kidney stones on the X-ray image.

Three dogs with implanted stones were placed on a conventional image converter table (Tridoros 5 S with image intensifier Sirecon Duplex 15/25 and X-ray tube Bi 125/30/50R) and X-rayed. In order to simulate the intervening water, water cushions of varying thickness (5-13 cm) were placed between the dog and the X-ray tube.

### 4.1.2 Integration of the X-ray locator

In constructing the location system the central beams of both X-ray systems were situated in a way that they intersected at the focus (f 2) of the semi-ellipsoid. The concretion can be placed exactly in the focal area by bringing the stone to the intersecting point of the beams. This point is marked by crosshairs in the middle of the image converter. The object to be photographed must be moved until it is situated in the middle of both systems.

The X-ray system used was the BV 22 from C. F. Müller Co (with automatic picture storage).

The X-ray planes are the first and second transverse section of the animal. Thereby the shock wave can be introduced from ventral to ventrolateral.

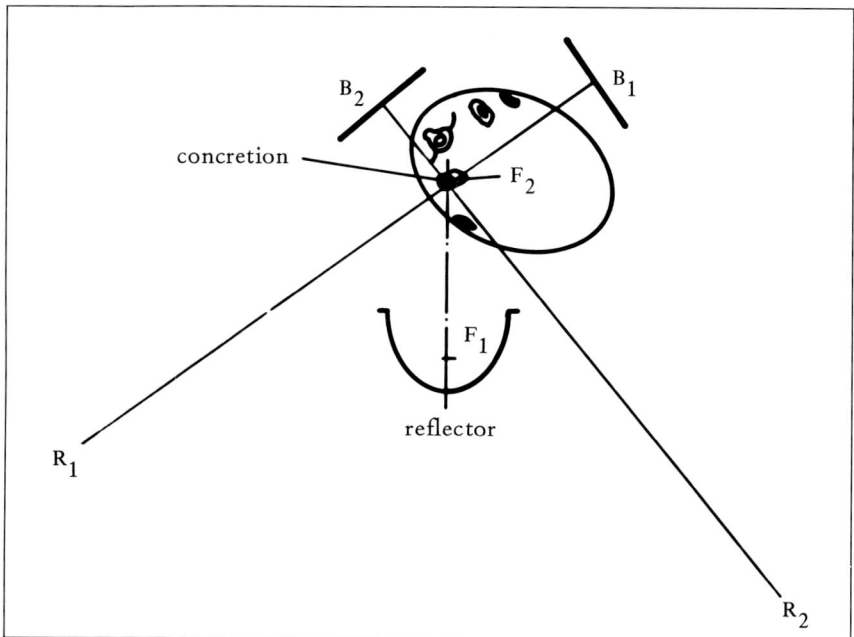

*Figure 42.* Sketch of the arrangement of the central beams of the X-ray location system.

### 4.1.3 Shock wave applicator

Following the plan of the prototypes used so far, this type is composed of three functional groups: the shock wave generator with ellipsoid and coupling tub, the X-ray location system and the positioning apparatus (figure 43). The shock wave generator and the ellipsoid are situated on a small adjustable support, so that the focal point of the ellipse can be adjusted with the location system. The underwater spark gap can be changed easily even with the bath full of water with the help of a sliding device and a cover on the ellipsoid.

Both X-ray systems (fig. 44) are mounted on swivel arms so that they may be moved up to an angle of 40° above the focal area. The image intensifiers and the X-ray tube are motorized on a movable slide, with which they can be moved towards or away from the focal point. Through a coupling, the distance between the X-ray tube and the image intensifier is held constant with any movement. The ellipsoid and the location system are adjustable within a geometrical exactness of 1 mm.

Based on the spacially fixed focus point of the underwater spark gap, the animal must be brought under the focal point by a device that can move in three dimensions. Therefore an automatic adjustment was built with which remotely controlled movement up to a speed of 2 mm/sec is possible.

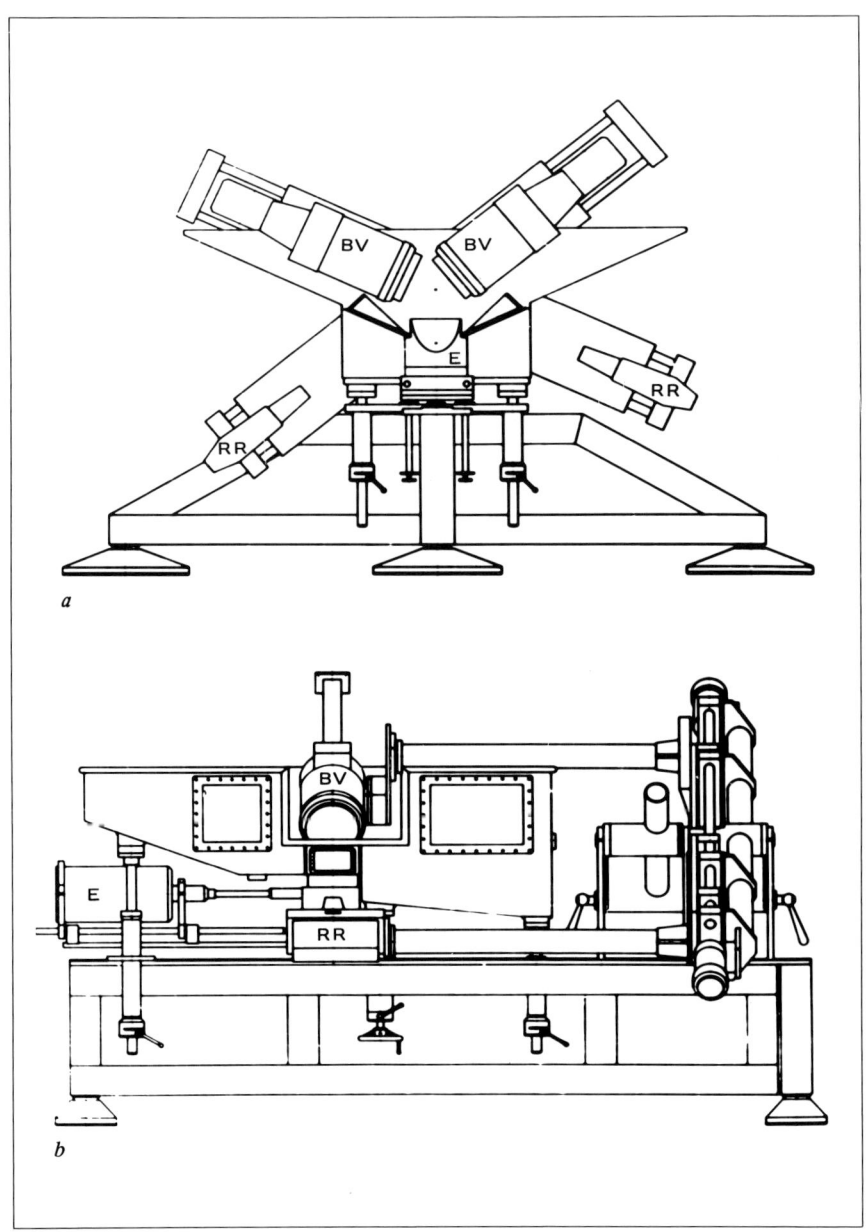

*Figure 43.* Schematic drawing of the study apparatus with integrated X-ray location system. BV = image intensifier, RR = X-ray tube, E = ellipsoid and underwater spark gap.
a) Front view.   b) side view.

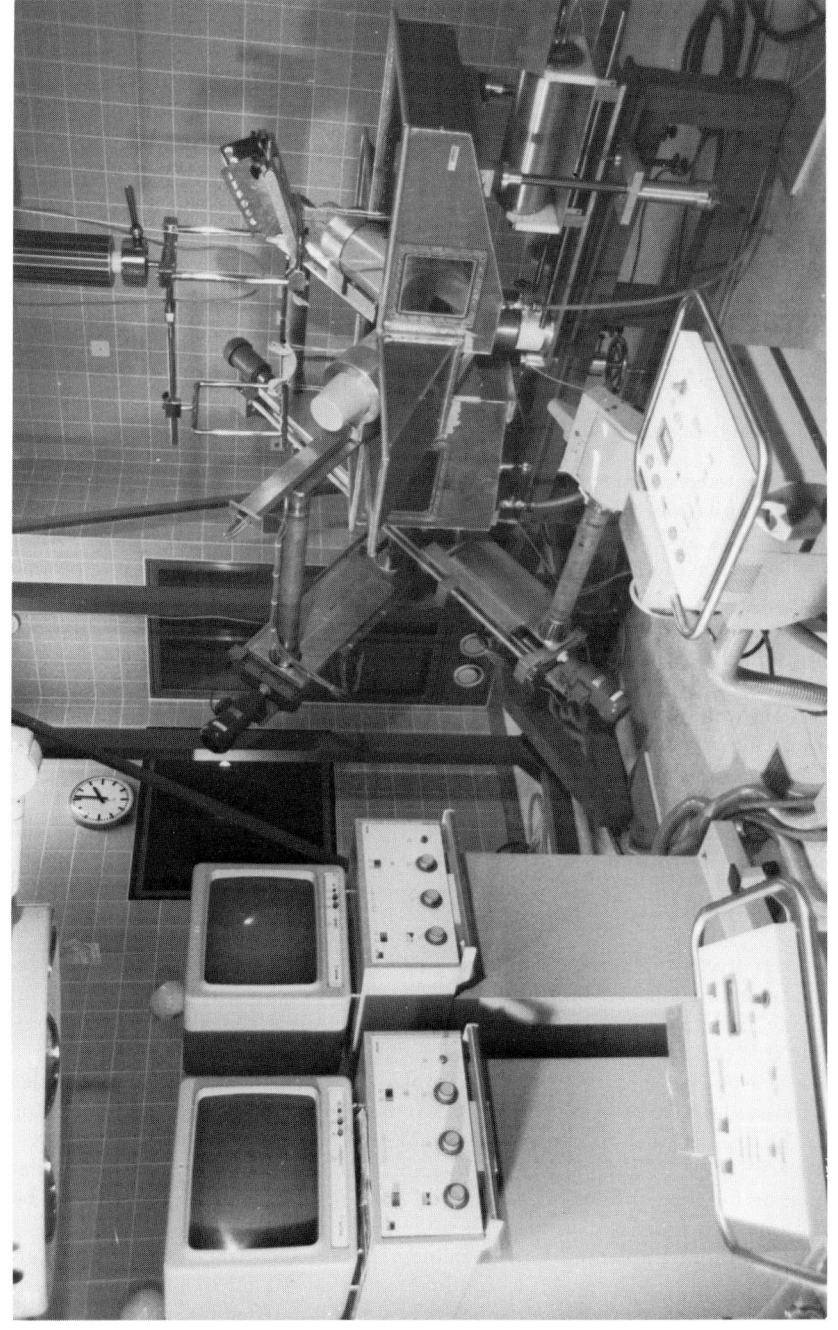

*Figure 44.* Photograph of the experimental apparatus with BV system and shock wave applicator.

*4.1.4 Changes of the shock wave energy/impulse series*

It was studied to what extent a change in pressure amplitude of the shock wave will influence the size of the fragments after exposure.

With a single shock wave exposure in the range of 2-3 kbar, larger, not spontaneously dischargeable stone fragments remained.

In in vitro studies a lowering of the pressure amplitude in the focal region from 2-3 kbar to 300 bar was achieved through a change in the condenser capacity from 2 microfarad to 20 nanofarad. In this energy range the in vitro study of shock wave exposure of human kidney stones was conducted, and the result was compared with the size of the pieces achieved through higher energy values.

*4.1.5 Animal studies*

a) Technical procedures

The anesthetized animal was, as in the previously described studies, placed after complete epilation of the abdominal area on its side in the positioning apparatus and then was moved into the tub above the ellipsoid. After this, the first manual gross adjustment until the stone was recognizable on one of the X-ray systems was done. By moving the image intensifier closer to the animal (so that the length of intervening water could be lessened), fine adjustment could be achieved by the X-ray control until the concretion was located in the crosshairs of both BV systems.

Taking into consideration exhalation, the shock wave treatment was begun in a series of impulses, whereby intermittent X-ray control verified the exact positioning in the focal point area.

When the treatment was completed, saline solution was administered intravenously and X-rays were taken in two planes for exact evaluation of the results of the destruction.

b) Study groups

Seventeen stone-implanted dogs were given 500 shock wave exposures. The results of the shock wave exposure immediately after the study and at three to four day intervals were monitored using X-rays until the animals were completely free of stones.

Shock wave exposure of non-stone-implanted dogs: Throughout the series of impulses, the total applied energy of the shock waves was held constant (given by the product of the shock number and the stored condenser energy). However in view of clinical application not even the least danger of organ degrading or function-influencing effects of a changed type of application can be tolerated.

Six dogs without implanted human kidney stones were placed in the study tub for shock wave exposure. After administration of 10 ml of 60 % megluminiothalamate (Conray 60) the renal pelvis could be identified by the image intensifiers and brought into the focus area. Then they received 500 shock wave exposures.

c) Experiments

Chemical studies: Before and after the study, as well as one and two weeks after shock wave exposure, blood samples were drawn from these animals for chemical monitoring, GOT, GPT, amylase, Hb, Hct, leukocytes, free plasma hemoglobin, Na (($Na^+$)), $K^+$, urea and creatinine were all analyzed.

Clearance study with $^{99m}$Tc-DMSA (dimercaptosuccinate): Before the experiment as well as 4 and 14 days thereafter, comparative clearance studies were done on each side of each animal with $^{99m}$technetium-dimercaptosuccinate ($^{99m}$Tc-DMSA) [52]. Four hours after intravenous injection of 1 ml $^{99m}$Tc-DMSA (1 mCi) the animals were placed before a scintillation camera for determination of the renal activity concentration on each side. With the help of "region-of-interest" techniques the absolute uptake of DMSA was counted for 30 seconds in each kidney. The DMSA uptake of the individual kidneys was determined directly after subtraction of the background (system: Intertechnik Company's Cine 200).

The evaluation of possible shock wave effects was accomplished by comparing the functional values of exposed and non-exposed kidney of the same test animal.

Histological studies: After completion of the clearance studies, the animals were subjected to a section. After macroscopic evaluation tissue samples from the lung, liver, kidney, pancreas, spleen, stomach, large and small intenstine, and ribs were taken.

## 4.2 Results

### 4.2.1 Effect of intervening water on X-ray location

With the described x-ray apparatus, concretions down to a size of 2-3 mm were discernible on the image converter. In this particular study arrangement the resolution was not altered by scattered radiation, even with a distance of 13 cm, so that the concretions were located with certainty (figure 45). Only with a very weakly contrasting concretion, there was difficulty of precise identification, e.g. when the stone was smaller than 5 mm.

### 4.2.2 Problems of pseudocavitation

By transmission of high compressive and tensile forces in the fluid a bubbling effect can occur (pseudocavitation) [41]. In the first experiments with 37 °C tap water there was such a build-up that the second shock wave was absorbed

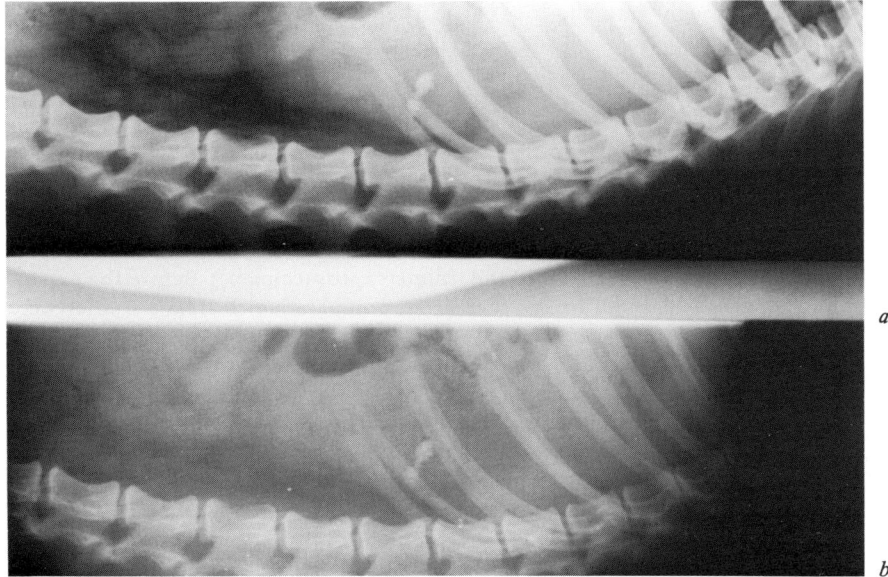

*Figure 45.* X-ray location experiment: Identification of an implanted kidney stone (a) without and (b) with a 13 cm long path through the intervening water.

so that there was not enough pressure at the focus to destroy the stones (figure 46). This bubbling depends on two parameters:

1. Composition in the water used as the coupling medium. Water containing carbon gives rise to a haze consisting of $CO_2$ bubbles.
2. Water temperature. The higher the temperature of the water the higher the partial pressure of physically dissolved gases. With application of water with lower temperature the partial pressure of the dissolved gases is lowered so that the application of the shock waves does not lead to a buildup of bubbles and therefore the absorption of the wave being transmitted is eliminated.

With the necessity of placing the experimental animal (or a patient) in the bath for the treatment the possibility of lowering the temperature in order to avoid the pseudocavitation effect is limited. Therefore the coupling fluid was degasified (distilled water) and was used at the still tolerable temperature of 30 °C. With these provisions the absorption effect of pseudocavitation was eliminated.

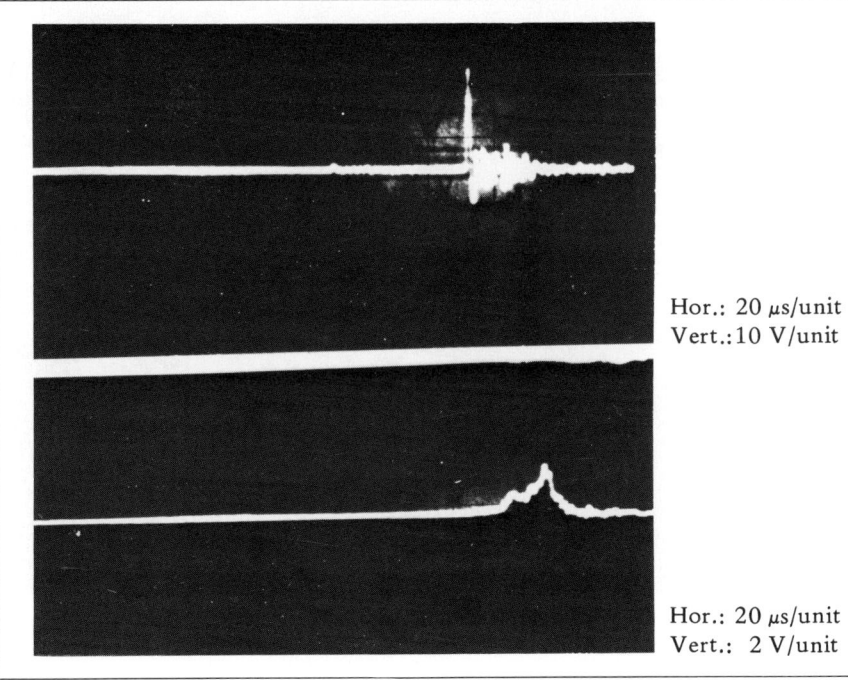

*Figure 46.* Pressure damping of the shock wave in water containing carbon and oxygen.

### 4.2.3 Kidney stone destruction with series impulses

A reduction of the shock wave energy from 700 joules to 25 joules demanded several shock wave exposures and led to a slower subdivision of the concretion with individual parts like particles of sand (figure 47).

In addition to a better disintegration capability, compared to a single impacting, of up to a 100 fold reduction of the pressure amplitude there is the advantage that the average shock wave energy is only 0.011 joule/cm$^2$, and therefore the acceleration of the individual particles is reduced to 0.4 m/s. Through this the stress on the surrounding tissues from the stone destruction is reduced.

### 4.2.4 Chemical studies after in vivo treatments

In table VI the values of various chemical parameters are given both before and after the shock wave exposure. No significant change is found after examination of the final values. Therefore no chemically discernible impact on the organs neighboring the kidney is found, such as the liver and the pancreas.

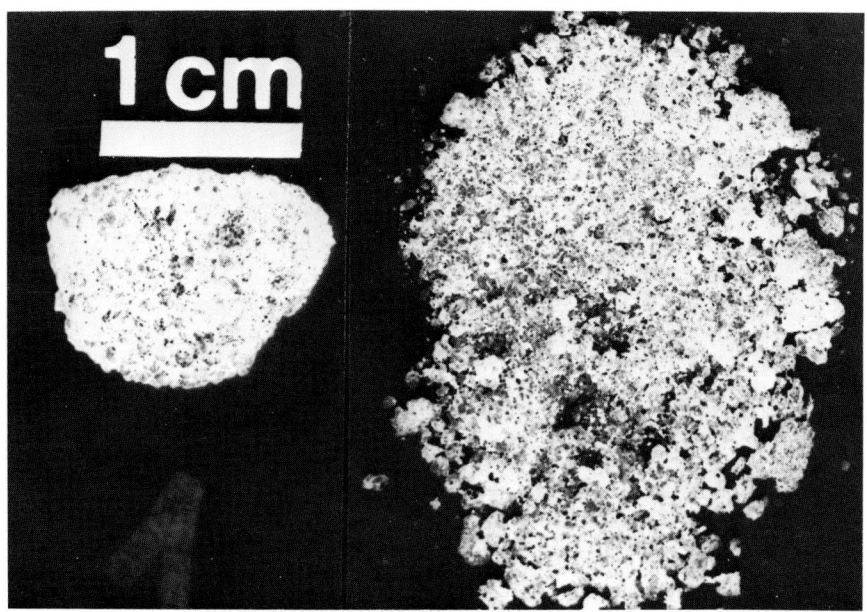

*Figure 47.* In vitro kidney stone destruction of a calcium oxalate stone. Number of exposures: 500.

### 4.2.5 Comparative clearance studies with $^{99m}Tc$-DMSA

In one of the six animals a difference in functional capability between the exposed right kidney and the unexposed left kidney was found. Table VII shows

*Table VI.* Laboratory values before and after 500 shock wave exposures

|  | before test | after shock wave exposure | 4 days after shock wave application | 10 days after shock wave application |
|---|---|---|---|---|
| GOT | 13.77± 2.14 | 17.30± 4.21 | 11.38± 1.48 | 11.68± 3.09 |
| GPT | 64.83±22.39 | 46.32± 7.98 | 40.20± 2.67 | 46.32± 7.73 |
| LDH | 104.50±34.39 | 127.30±13.18 | 80.40±12.52 | 70.68± 2.06 |
| AP | 139.40±27.80 | 152.90±23.00 | 188.20±29.30 | 173.30±46.07 |
| a-Amylase | 1.47± 0.16 | 1.48± 1.49 | 1.20± 0.10 | 1.38± 0.20 |
| Potassium mval/1 | 4.50± 1.46 | 4.39± 1.33 | 3.93± 2.57 | 4.45± 1.29 |
| Sodium mval/1 | 146.80± 3.38 | 152.20± 1.33 | 146,70± 2.35 | 148.30± 1.08 |
| Creatine mg% | 0.80± 0.09 | 0.76± 0.10 | 0.80± 0.06 | 0.74± 0.08 |
| Urea-N mg% | 12.95± 1.65 | 10.76± 0.49 | 13.37± 0.90 | 12.97± 1.30 |

*Table VII.* Behavior of the clearance values of the shock wave exposed right kidney, 4 and 14 days after trial in % of the initial value and quotient of the right and left kidney

|  | before exposure | | 4 days after exposure | | 14 days after exposure | |
|---|---|---|---|---|---|---|
|  | r. kidney initial value in % | ratio r:l kidney | r. kidney in % of initial value | ratio r:l kidney | r. kidney in % of initial value | ratio r:l kidney |
| DMSA 1 | 100 % | 1.22 | 107 % | 1.34 | 91 % | 1.02 |
| DMSA 2 | 100 % | 1.17 | 113 % | 1.56 | 92 % | 1.04 |
| DMSA 3 | 100 % | 1.13 | 120 % | 1.78 | 123 % | 1.86 |
| DMSA 4 | 100 % | 1.63 | 94 % | 1.38 | 102 % | 1.70 |
| DMSA 5 | 100 % | 1.70 | 100 % | 1.70 | 105 % | 1.78 |
| DMSA 6 | 100 % | 1.38 | 77 % |  | 135 % | 1.86 |
|  | 100 % | 1.37±0,09 | 100.2±7.6 | 1.44±0.13 | 106±8.15 | 1.50±0.19 |

the quotients obtained from the clearance percentages of the right and left kidneys and their changes after shock wave exposure in percent of the initial values. There was no lessening of the activity concentration within the boundaries of the kidney area observed in any experiment, as would have to be expected in the case of degradation of function or destruction within the boundaries of the kidney. Figure 48 shows the scintigrams obtained from a study animal both before and after the shock wave exposure.

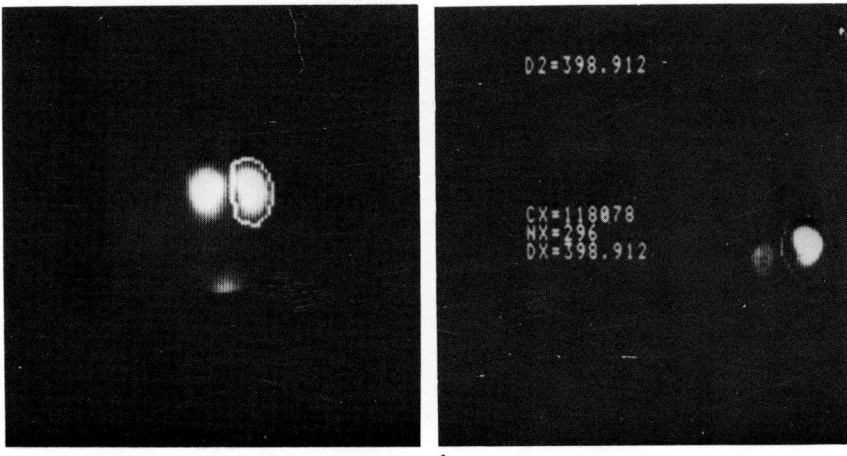

*a*        *b*

*Figure 48.* Equal activity concentrations in both kidneys: Picture before (a) and after (b) the study. The treated kidney is on the right. The pictures are taken on the dorsal side.

### 4.2.6 Histological evaluation

Also in this experimental group neither macroscopic nor microscopic pathological changes were seen. None of the studied organs showed changes which could be caused by a traumatizing effect of the shock wave. In figure 49 there is a histological section of the kidney after 500 shock wave exposures.

### 4.2.7 In vivo stone destruction

Altogether 17 stone carrying animals were subjected to a 500 shock wave exposure; after the experiments regular X-ray monitoring was conducted. In 13 of these animals, a spontaneous discharge of all concretion could be achieved. In none of the animals either during or after the experiment was any negative impact on their overall aspect observed that could be traced to the shock wave exposure. This is verified by the results of the histological studies of the kidneys and the surrounding tissue. Also, no lesions of the right lower lung lobe were seen when the X-ray locator was employed to conduct the kidney stone destruction - either with macroscopic or microscopic means - as it was observed with the screen exposure.

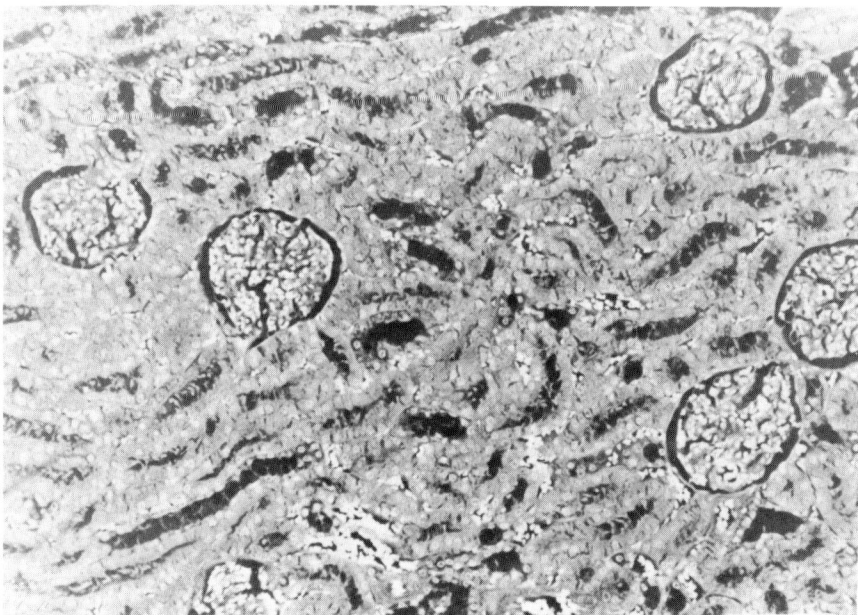

*Figure 49.* Histological section of a dog kidney after 500 shock wave exposures (100 x enlargement).

The time needed for the complete discharge of the concretion fragments was between 1 and 4 weeks. It should be mentioned that, for technical reasons, a "stone expulsion therapy" is not possible with research animals over such a period of time.

In three animals a second shock wave treatment was conducted 14 days later to further reduce the larger concretion fragments remaining in the kidney cavity. Through this additional exposure 2 animals were freed of their stones after 14 days. In four animals, no complete stone freedom could be accomplished. Three of the animals, being brought into the 30 °C water bath showed a pronounced hyperventilation with strong exhalation, so that it was not possible to keep the stone in the exact focus because of the extremely heavy breathing. Therefore, these were declared mistrials because only a fragment of the shock wave bombarded the stone.

Figures 50a-c show the radiograms before, immediately after and four weeks after the exposure of the animal. Even though the exposure led to complete disintegration of the concretion so that the fragments could be discharged (figure 50b), one can see in a later radiogram (4 weeks later) a dust-like film on the renal pelvis (figure 50c). A histological study of the kidney revealed that small fragments of the concretion had deposited in fibrin causing edema of the epithelium of the urinary tract resulting in pronounced pyelonephritis. In none of the examined sections were any of these dust-like particles found in the epithelium of the urinary tract.

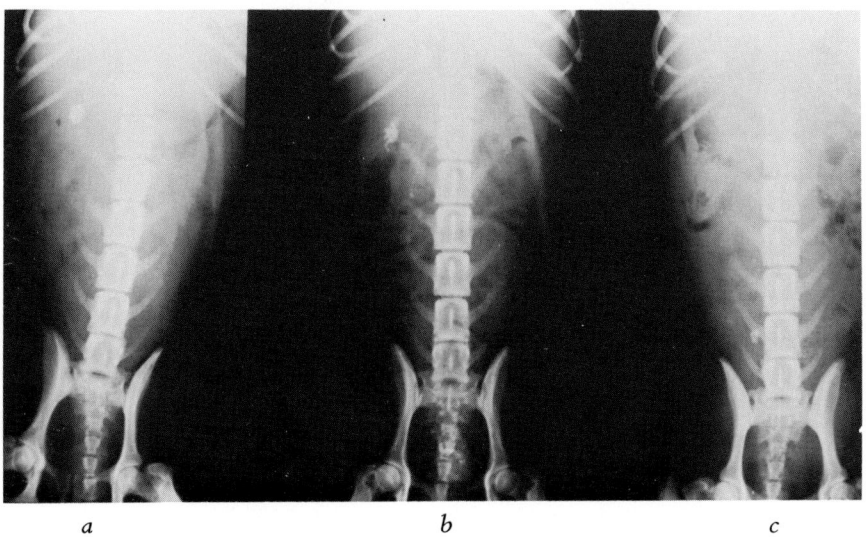

*Figure 50.* Overall view radiogram before (a), immediately after (b) and 4 weeks after (c) shock wave exposure.

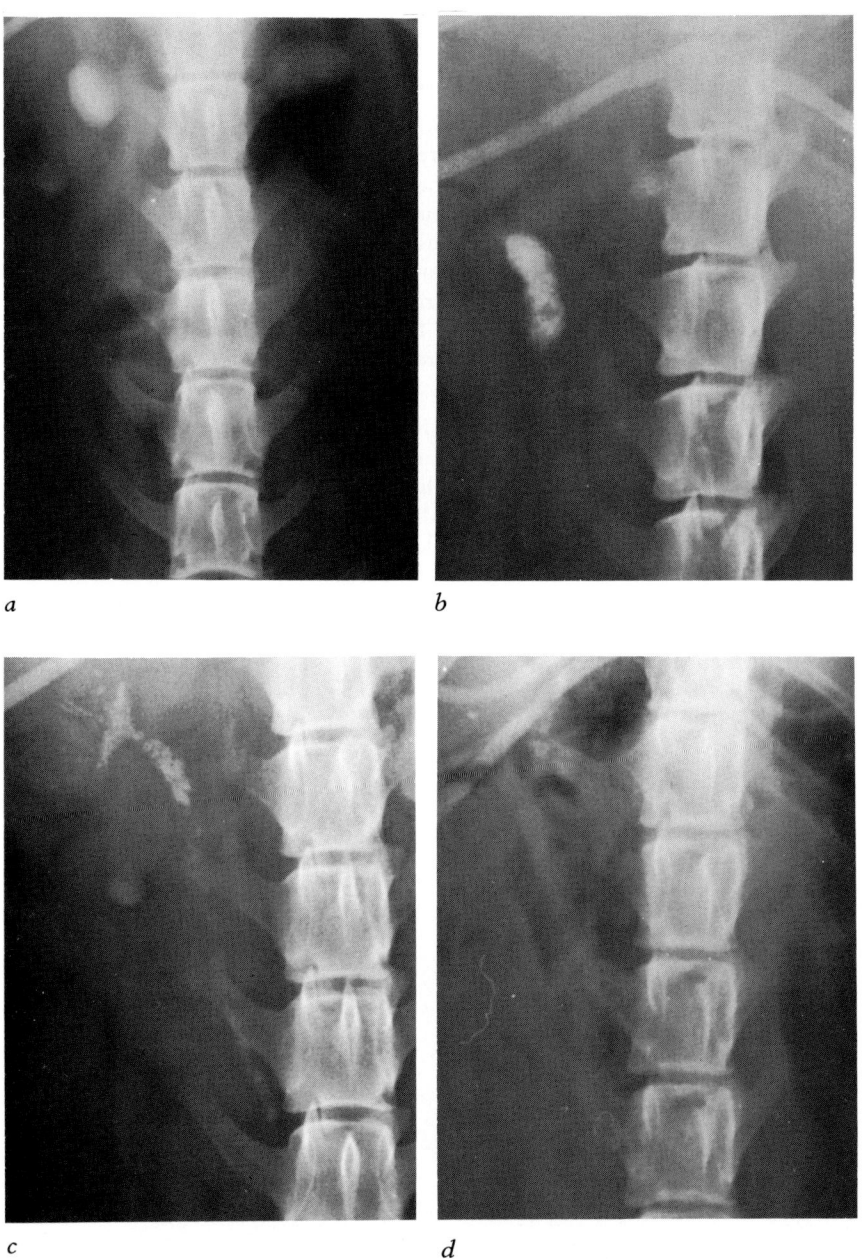

*Figure 51.* Monitoring after shock wave exposure: a) before, b) + c) immediately after and d) 14 days after treatment.

Figures 51a-d show the X-ray monitoring of a study for contact-free kidney stone destruction. After a 500 shock wave exposure, a pronounced divergence and contrast non-uniformity of the concretion can be compared with the radiogram before treatment. A fluid load to induce a forced diuresis shows the treatment effects much more clearly.

Figure 52 shows that only two hours after exposure a spontaneous discharge of the pellets of the reduced kidney stone has begun. Freedom from stones can be documented by X-ray only 7 days after treatment.

Additional examples are shown in figure 53 and figure 54. In both cases freedom from stones was documented ten days after treatment.

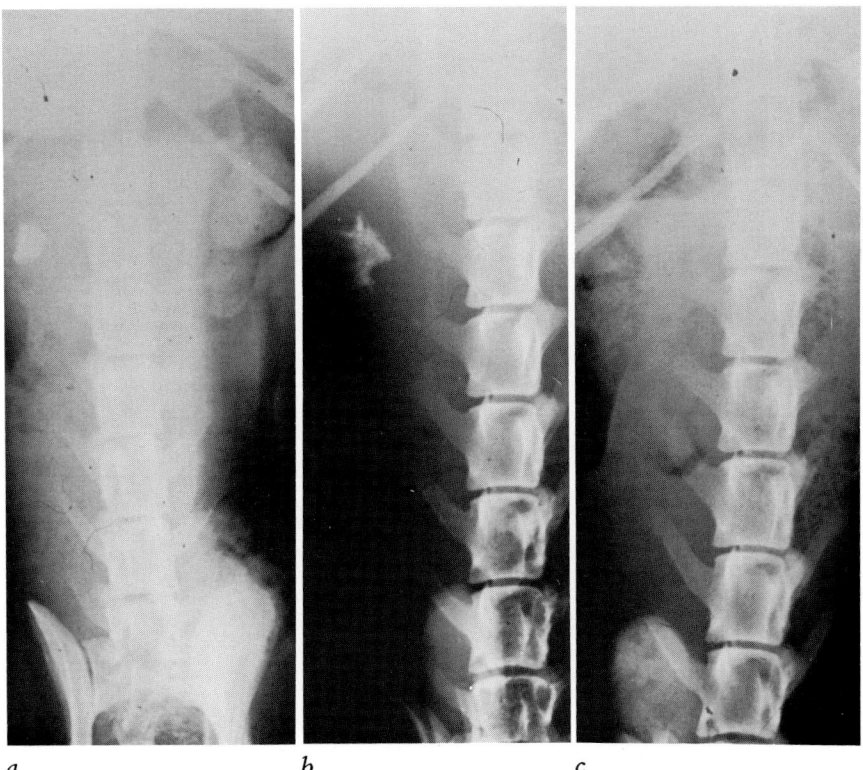

a    b    c

*Figure 52.* X-ray monitoring a) before b) immediately after and c) 7 days after shock wave exposure.

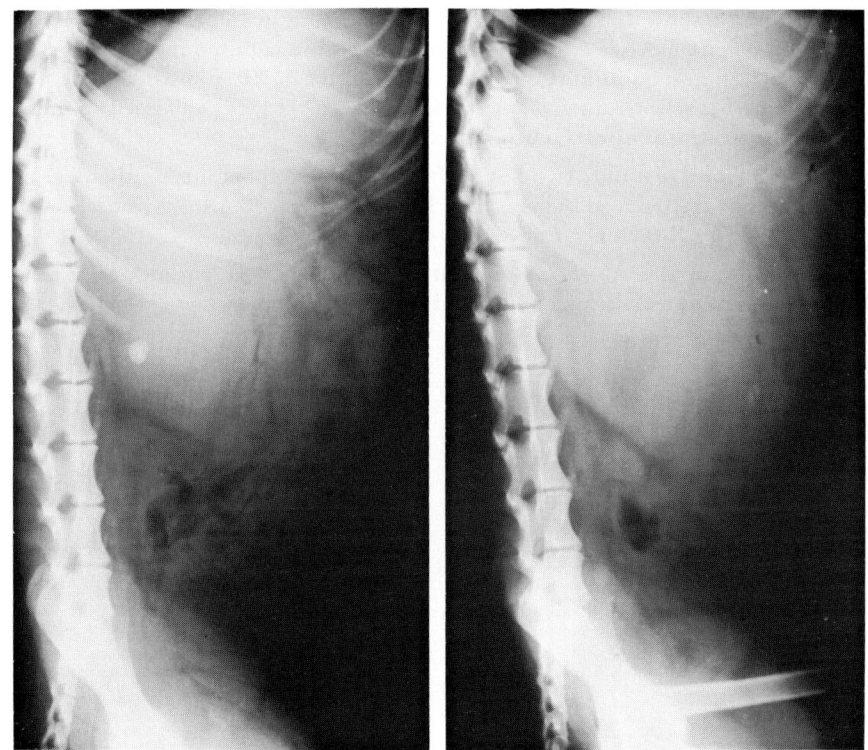

*Figure 53.* Radiogram before and 10 days after shock wave exposure.

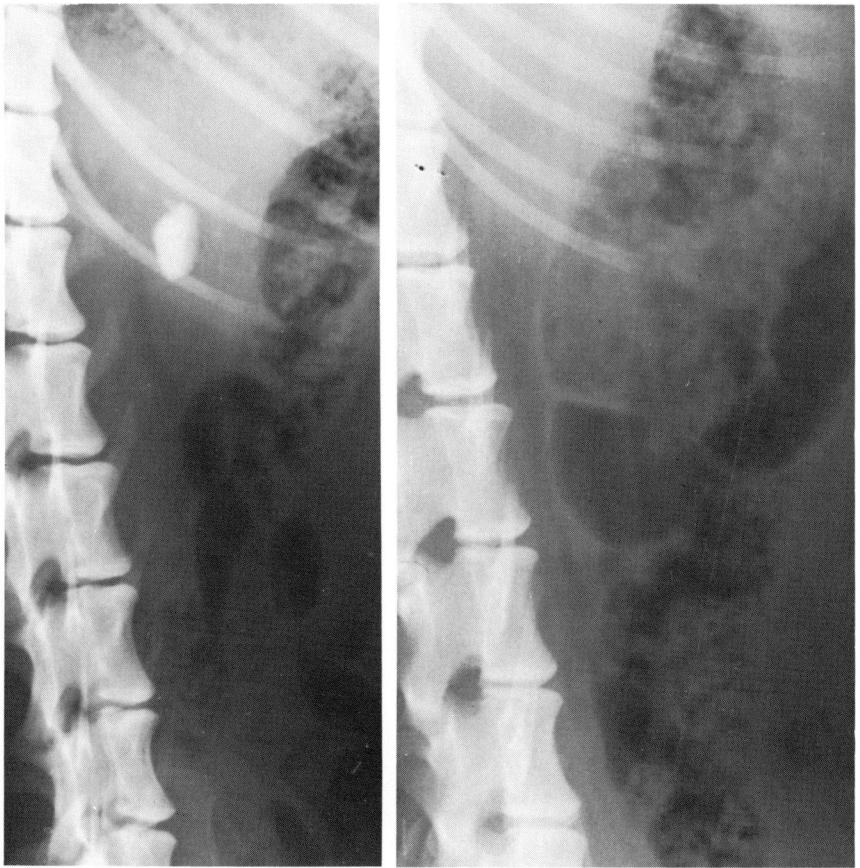

*Figure 54.* Radiogram before and 10 days after shock wave exposure.

# Discussion

On the basis of the described tests and results it was proven for the first time that the transmission of high energy shock waves through living organisms could be accomplished without recognizable tissue or functional degradation of the organic system. One of the basic requirements is that there be no interfaces of structures having different acoustical impedances which can affect the transmission of the shock waves. There is no physical transformation experienced by the underwater generated and conducted shock wave in living tissue which contains approximately 70 % water, so that even pressure amplitudes of 3-4 kbar can be tolerated, and this also applies to vital bone structure.

The fact that erythrocytes are partially hemolyzed seems to contradict this basic behavior and can only be explained by a certain amount of already dying, old erythrocytes, existing already in each blood sample. The membrane stability of the erythrocytes or nucleated cells change with age.

If you consider that even by applying the shock wave onto the vascularized organs and vessels, this hemolyzing action is only limited to a focal range of 1.5 cm$^3$ and afterwards a systematic distribution of the freed hemoglobin takes place to the complete blood volume, it is not surprising that no increase of the free plasma hemoglobin in the peripheral blood can be determined. Only after a 500 repetitive shock wave application, a slight increase of plasma hemoglobin and LDH was seen immediately after the experiment which was reversed after two hours and is explained by the traumatizing of erythrocytes.

By excluding the tissue damaging effects, the main requirement for the therapeutic application of shock waves was met. The first application area chosen was the contact-free destruction of kidney stones, though other applications can be imagined. In the work presented here the individual development steps are described which led to this result.

After the necessary preliminary studies in order to clarify the biological tolerance, the technical development of the apparatus was approached, with which human kidney stones of any composition in specially developed animal models were destroyed with accuracy and consistency to such an extent that they were reduced to spontaneously dischargeable fragments.

A difficult problem was the location of the concretion in living tissue, which was necessary to bring the shock wave into the focus, which is identical to the location of the kidney stone.

In the beginning, two ultrasound transducers which were integrated into the shock wave ellipsoid were used in order to perform the locating. This procedure was not useful because of the superposition of the ultrasonic echoes which made a certain location of the concretion impossible. Therefore, a control over the destruction and discharge of the fragments was not possible. Nevertheless, the mistrials with the ultrasonic location and its results were described in section three of this work, because only a "negative success" of this study justified the use of the subsequently used X-ray location procedure with its great expense.

After the described in vivo and in vitro studies, with the exception of a not important hemolysis showing no signs of cell or tissue damage, there was no sound reason to avoid clinical use of the shock wave device. In spite of this clear statement the danger of tissue damage needs to be discussed further because of its fundamental importance.

*The danger of tissue damage*

With the developed trial apparatus shock waves were generated at the focal point of a hollow ellipsoid, which were propagated to a second focal point located in the tissue having a maximum pressure of 0.3 - 3.0 kbar in the focal area (volume = 1.5 cm$^3$). With the latest apparatus used in the study, instead of a single shock wave, a series of shock waves of lower energy could be applied, where in the second focal area pressures of only 400 bars appear. By ignoring the physical law that only tissue-damaging tensile and compressive stresses can be established by transmission of such shock waves when phase boundaries between differing acoustical impedances are crossed, for example, the air in the alveolus, the lack of tissue damage in this study can be explained by the fact that only in the focal region is so high a pressure established.

Before reaching the focal area, the shock waves reflected by the hollow ellipsoid have only slight pressure and diverge after their convergence at the second focal point as a set of rays (see figure 55). It is only a very small area in which theoretically dangerous pressures can build. But only when there is a boundary between substances of differing acoustical impedance in this small area will compressive and tensile stresses develop which destroy the structure.

The "trick", consisting of discharging a spark gap in a hollow ellipsoid thus allowing the generated shock waves to concentrate in the second focus, does not only have the value of creating an especially high energy density but also has the aim of minimizing the pressures which can develop outside the desired focal area. Nevertheless, it should be mentioned that even with the transmission of a diffuse high energy pressure wave, structures with another acoustical den-

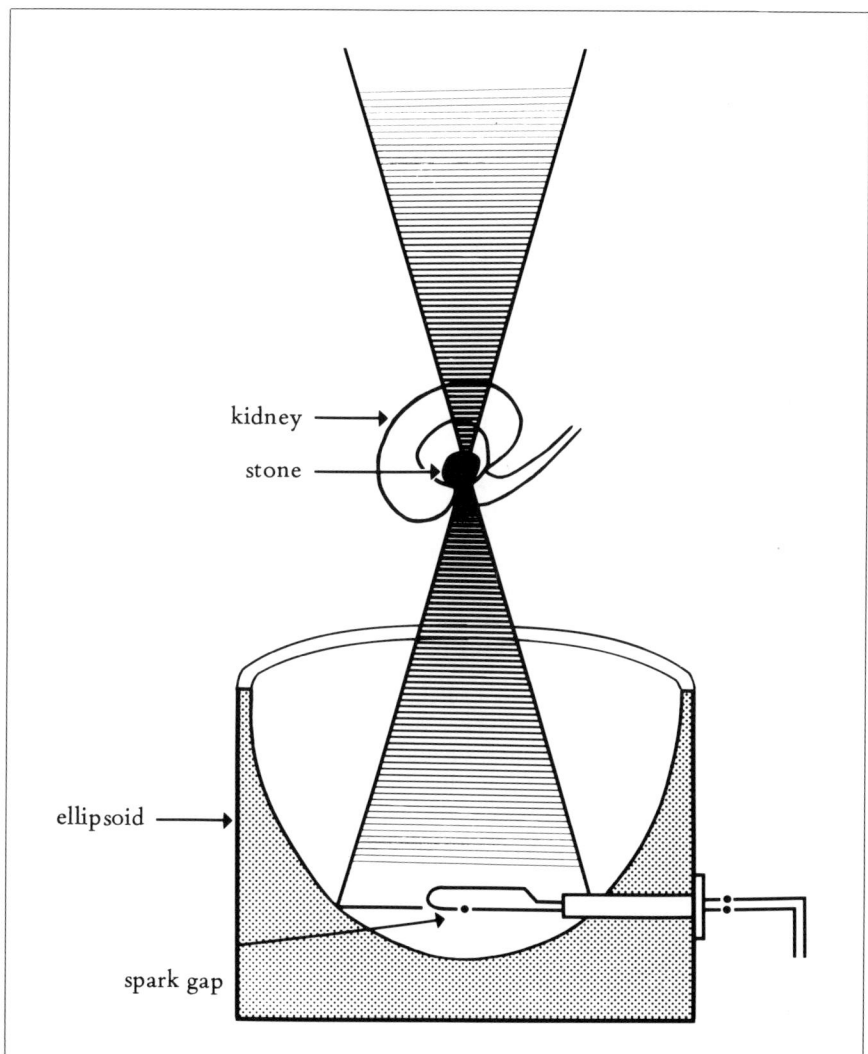

*Figure 55.* Schematic representation of pressure transmission of shock wave exposure. The density of the screen compares with the approximate pressure density of the transmitting pressure as it moves through the tissue.

sity can be destroyed, and that the focusing alone does not necessarily cause a destructive effect. And this is not only present in the physical principles of shock wave physics but also can be shown through the presented studies:

If a shock wave with a pressure of 2-3 kbars is moving through an experimental animal whose opposite body side is not covered by water, there will be slight tissue damage at the interface of the tissue and air. It can be recognized by the petechial bleeding in the affected areas. This occurs in spite of the fact that only relatively low pressures are obtained outside the focal point because of the divergence of the waves. The applicability of the method depends on the fact that the acoustical properties of the tissue medium do not appreciably differ from water. To avoid tissue damage the most important and uncompromisable prerequisite is therefore the maintenance of a transmission medium as identical as possible.

How dangerous shock wave exposure can be, when this basic rule is not attended, is shown by the studies of shock wave exposure on the thoracic region of a rat, where it resulted in extensive lung damage. The great difference in the acoustical properties of air as opposed to tissue in the alveoli of the lung creates a great number of acoustical interfaces, where part of the shock wave is reflected with a phase reversal, so that a tensile stress is created on the membranes which greatly exceeds its tensile strength.

These results led to two demands for shock wave application: one was to work with the smallest possible and therefore most clearly delimited focal region and also the demand for a more reliable method for location of the concretion when using shock waves in the region of the lung for the destruction of kidney stones.

The same behavior as in the lung can theoretically also occur when the shock wave comes to the gas-filled intestine. Although in none of the in vivo studies macroscopic and histologic damages could be determined with eventual clinical application, caution must be taken that there is no distension of the intestine. Even if the transmission of shock waves through the gas-filled intestine results in no damage, in order to be of clinical use, this condition must be avoided, lest reflection of the shock waves from this region of the intestine prevent a sufficient buildup of pressure at the site of stone destruction. For clinical application the intestine must be prepared by a special roughage-free diet.

The question of which pressure must be employed in order to destroy kidney stones of various compositions was studied by *Häusler* (Institute of Physics at the University of Saarbrücken). The strength parameters which he found are assembled in table VIII.

The necessary static pressure lies around 80 bars while the tensile strength is considerably lower. In designing such a shock wave apparatus there was actually no need to go to such intensities which created pressures of 300 bars in the focal area. Unfortunately, this was not technically possible, because for consistent generation the necessary spark gap voltage must be at least 12-15 kV for discharge, and in the employed system this created a pressure at the second focus of 300 bars. To examine the biological tolerance, shock waves with a pressure of up to 3-4 kbar were used to determine the dangers should such pressures ever be indicated for a clinical application.

*Table VIII.* Stability values of the kidney stones

| Composition | $P_Z$ (bar) | $P_D$ (bar) |
|---|---|---|
| Magnesium ammonium phosphate | 6 | 80 |
| Tricalcium phosphate + uric acid | 6 | 40 |
| Tricalcium phosphate | – | 48 |
| Uric acid | 18 | – |
| Ca-oxalate | 11 | – |
| Gallstone | 4-10 | 22-32 |

For example, that could be the case if other stones need to be destructed at a greater distance from the shock wave device where of course a semi-ellipsoid with a wider focus must be used. If with a 6 cm tissue transmission the shock wave already received a damping of 10-20 % (see fig. 14), situations are clearly forseeable, for instance for the more corpulent individual, where the shock wave needs to be focused on the concretion at a distance of 12 cm. It is not only theoretically but also practically important to know that pressures which were actually discussed in the study as not necessary were tolerated when all other precautions were followed.

After the in vivo tests with the lymphocyte culture had shown that the proliferative quality of such sensitive cells cannot be influenced, the only remaining possibility of tissue damage during the application might be a lesion of the endothelium of the collecting system. As shown in many discussions the layman thinks of an explosive separation of the exposed kidney stones where the fragments are shot into the endothelium. But this is not possible because, on the one hand, the shock creates pressure on the surface where it enters the stone and, on the other hand, creates tension when it is reflected from the back wall. Both forces operate centripetally so that the concretion crumbles rather than splits. On the other hand, the acceleration of the fragments of the concretion lasts only for a microsecond so that even if the forces are great the momentum is still unappreciable. Indeed, with cooperative work with the physicists of **Dornier System** in these studies, only a slight dispersing motion of the fragments of the concretion could be measured, and the maximum obtainable kinetic energy of a single particle was found to be $2 \times 10^{-3}$ joules, which compares with the kinetic energy of a falling raindrop. In the last developed apparatus with which only a focal pressure of 300-600 bar could be achieved, the created kinetic energy is only a tenth of this value and even if very sharp fragments are produced, it is unimaginable that there would be any damage to the endothelium.

Finally, one further possibility of damage was considered, that the fragments have very sharp corners which can reach the ureter and not only cause ureteral colic but also damage to the urothelium. Even though this was not observed in the animal studies, the possibility cannot be excluded and the method must be verified clinically.

*The stone model*

In the preclinical tests of kidney stone destruction with shock waves, the need arises for an experimental model using animals which is sufficiently comparable to the human situation. There is no animal known which develops kidney stones with any regularity nor were experimental methods known for inducing stones in the animals with any certainty in an appropriate amount of time [51,54]. Even when stones were induced by prolonged special diets, the location could not be influenced and the concretions that did appear were in the bladder and the ureter but only seldom in the kidney cavity. In addition, there is a special problem of stone induction by special diet, since the inducing substances must be given in such high concentrations that they themselves can cause toxic kidney damage. Therefore an evaluation of the damaging influence of shock wave application would be limited. From these considerations there was only one development of the animal experiments which are recorded here for the first time, where human kidney stones of different compositions and sizes by a two step operation procedure were placed in the kidney cavity of the dog [27,27].

The advantages of this model are obvious: kidney stones which actually occur in clinical situations could be studied, and these could be selected according to the size and composition for a series of studies. The implantation of the larger kidney stones was only possible when the collecting system was delated in the first operative procedure by a ligature of the ureter. This was not a disadvantage because after reimplantation of the ureter following stone implantation the ureter reverted to its normal "dog size" after 14 days. It was even tighter than a normal human ureter. The anatomical study conditions were therefore related to the spontaneous discharge capability, even more unfavorable than in a person.

It can be assumed that, since in dog models the stone fragments were discharged spontaneously, that it will be much easier in humans. But such a conclusion is not justified for the following reasons: In none of the cases was any pain or colic observed either during stone implantation or after shock wave exposure, even when fragments were lodged in the ureter (this was proven by X-ray). The behavior patterns of the animals were known to the scientists and the animals' keepers. In each case they were able to recognize when the animals were in pain either post operationem or because of some complication and were familiar with their reactions to the administered medication. It therefore raises the question of whether dogs for whom kidney stones are extremely rare - with the exception of dalmations - have evolved general receptors in the ureter which lead to colic pain similar to humans. The regularly observed spontaneous discharge of the kidney stones or their fragments after shock wave exposure can therefore be more easily accomplished in dogs than in humans because the ureter spasms were either slight or nonexistent.

*Location system*

For the application of a shock wave therapy in a clinical treatment the exact location of the concretion is an absolute prerequisite. The focal area of 1.5 cm$^3$ where the destruction of concretions is exclusively possible requires an exact locating. On the other hand, as the study showed, any exposure of the lung must be avoided. Therefore a screen exposure as was used in the experiments is unacceptable in the clinic.

Principally there are two methods available for location which can be discussed: either the spark gap and the location system - ultrasonic or X-ray - can be moved in two planes over the fixed experimental animal or the other way around, hollow ellipsoid with location system stationary and the animal movable in three dimensions. The latter system was selected out of purely practical considerations. It is technically easier to construct an apparatus which will move the animal and not the ultrasonic transducer or the later employed adjustable X-ray system.

The first studies for location of the stones were conducted with ultrasonic for two reasons:

1. The acoustical propagation of ultrasound and the shock waves follow the same physical laws.
2. The use of ultrasonic is, from the medical standpoint, completely uncomplicated and without danger for the patient and represents no additional load to clinical personnel.

Beside these plausible, theoretical advantages for the use of ultrasound, the first studies already showed that a clear echo structure of the stones even in parameter-free in vitro systems was possible only down to a size of 5 mm. Also with in vivo application in patients a sonographic identification of stones as small as 8 mm was possible only in 30 %. Additional difficulties were found in the animals because it was necessary to perform the locating through perirenal scar tissue resulting from the surgery. This resulted in reflection zones and artefacts with created superposition making recognition of the stone even more difficult. A further disadvantage of the integrated ultrasonic system is that even when there was a clear identification of the stone, it was in no case possible to monitor the progress of the destruction during the shock wave exposure.

Therefore the only alternative was to use X-ray scanning real-time representation to conduct the experiments. The difficulties of designing such a device, which were substantial at the outset, are not completely presented here. One of the disadvantages arising from the requirements placed on the X-ray location system by the shock wave application was that the only way to gather the necessary stereoscopic information for projective image representation consisted in the use of a second independent image converter system. The second X-ray system had to be placed in such a way that its central beam cuts the central beam of the first apparatus in the focal point of the ellipsoid. Therefore, the exact focal position of the concretion must be established so that the stone lies in the crossing point of both central beams.

Therefore, a precise location of the stone was possible down to a size of 1-2 mm where such a location had been impossible even under the most favorable conditions using ultrasound. There was no difficulty of establishing a successful monitoring during the shock wave exposure.

*Discharge capability of the concretion fragments*

The possibility of damage to biological systems has been excluded by the previous studies. Therefore from the clinical point of view this method is viable. The question of the discharge capability of the concretion fragments after exposure remained a slight problem. As already discussed, transferring the techniques of shock wave application to humans from dogs, even regarding our successes, cannot be made without adequate caution. But the fact remains that in the animal studies the anatomical conditions were more disadvantageous than in clinical situations, even though not everything is known about a comparison of the functional system of stone discharge of the dog and of the human.

It was already clear at the beginning of the tests that for clinical application the concretion fragments needed to be very small. Studies about the spontaneous discharge capability were helpful to quantify the demands of obtaining the smallest possible fragments. *Wax* and *Frank* [97] discovered in their patients that 83 % of the stones up to a diameter of 4 mm and 36 % of the stones of a diameter from 5-10 mm are capable of being discharged spontaneously. *Sandgard* [78, 79] found similiar results where a 93 % spontaneous discharge of concretions of up to 4 mm could be observed. 53 % of patients were freed of their stones through conventional therapy with stones of 4-6 mm.

Consequently, these findings warrant a clinical application of contact-free kidney stone destruction only when it is possible to reduce the concretions to fragments of less than 4 mm in diameter [46, 35]. This goal was not possible with the apparatus described in part three. Even though repeated application (5-10 times) of high energy shock waves (2-3 kbars) led to a destruction of the stone, it did not accomplish destruction of the individual pieces down to a size of 1-4 mm. Discharge of larger fragments will certainly lead to a blockage of urinary flow and this makes the spontaneous discharge of smaller pieces impossible, ultimately requiring some kind of operative procedure for their removal.

Only the development of the apparatus for generating a salvo of shock waves with low pressure amplitude brought about a pronounced improvement. Therefore it was possible to destroy the stone into pieces so that they were not larger than 1-2 mm. Fragments of this size can be spontaneously discharged according to the most current clinical experience. Even though the concretion fragments have very sharp edges there should be little difficulty in passing them because they are so small. After shock wave exposure, this patient can be compared with a patient who suffers from small ureter stones. The patient can then be subjected to conventional therapies which shorten the discharge time and relieve the patient showing colic-like symptoms. Such auxiliary therapy with spasmolysants and forced diuresis will represent a standard part in the therapeutic regime to this shock wave procedure. These aftertreatments were simply not possible with experimental animals for technical reasons. A single injection of a spasmolysant and 300 ml of physiological saline solution did lead to the more rapid discharge of the stone in the dog, which is conclusively shown in figure 56. The therapy which was begun immediately after the study led to an almost instant flushing of the stone through the natural pathway. It is therefore to be hoped that, in consequent follow-up treatment of the patient, the four week long process of discharging the fragments can be shortened considerably.

*Clinical application and indication*

With the morbidity rate of 2-3 % of the total population, nephrolithiasis can be compared to the frequency of manifest diabetes [2, 38, 82]. Therefore it is not surprising that 70 years ago an intensive research began [70, 80] to find out the fundamentals of kidney stone disease. Results of this research are mirrored in the varying theories [3, 11-13, 18, 31, 72, 86, 93], but as so often happens in medical research, it can not be concealed that the actual mechanism has not been found. This means, on the other hand, that a preventitive therapy of the urinary stone disease or an effective metaphylaxis is not always possible.

Considering that there is an approximately 50-70 % recurrence rate for stone patients [87, 25] there is the frightening aspect for the patient that the operation can only take care of the symptoms to avoid secondary damage.

There are limits to this symptomatic operative therapy. If the operative removal of a "simple" stone is a relatively uncomplicated procedure [2, 9, 99] it would be quite different for the first and the second recurrence. *Hartung et al.* [38] show that the first operation has a nephrectomy rate of 11.5 %. This number is an example how the clinical risks increase with several operations on the kidney. If you further consider that there is a pronounced peak of kidney stone disease for people between 30 and 40 years [8, 9, 99] it is obvious that with such a relatively young patient the organs should be treated with great care meaning that atraumatic, non-operative removal of the stone should be striven for. The possibility exists according to the presented results to reach

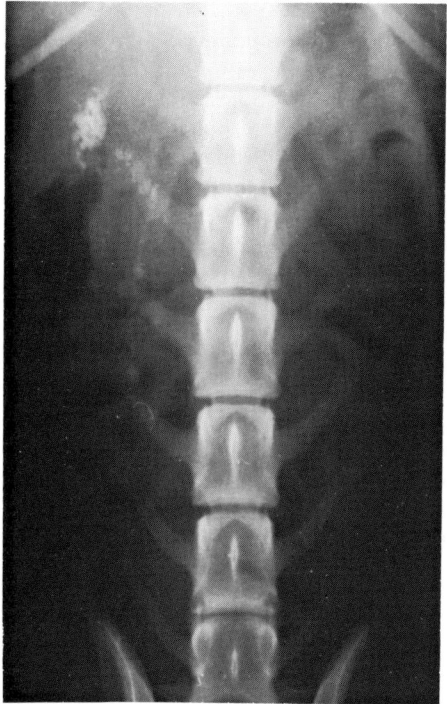

*Figure 56.* Concretion discharge after giving 300 ml of physiological saline solution immediately after shock wave esposure.

the goal of applying contact-free kidney stone destruction to some of the patients.

The range of indication of this method in the clinical application can only be speculated at this point based on the presented animal tests and will be shown after the first series of human application.

In principle there are two areas of application:

1. the destruction of solitary kidney and ureter stones to obtain a spontaneous discharge of the fragments;
2. a pre-operative shock wave application for patients with staghorn stones or calyx stones trapped in the renal pelvis by a stenosis, in order to eliminate the functional interference and organic degradation caused by the stone removal through the parenchyma by nephrotomies.

As has been frequently mentioned, there is with each spontaneous discharge the theoretical possibility of intermittent partial urinary blockage because of small fragments. Such an occurence will be tolerated by the patient and does not lead to complications. On the other hand, even a brief obstruction of the urinary flow can cause infected urine and a potentially life-threatening urosepsis.

Therefore the application of the method to infected stone carriers is limited, until unequivocal results concering the action of stone flushing in the patient completely eliminate this danger.

The basis for the application of this method is the discharge of the concretion fragments in a natural way. This possibility is limited per se by anatomically caused hindrances to the flow, for instance, in ureteral stenosis or stricture. In these cases, an appropriate therapy does not only eliminate the concretion, it also restores undisturbed flow conditions. Otherwise there is a high possibility of a quick stone recurrency.

Another often asked question, which could not be answered by the animal tests, is the painfulness of a shock wave exposure. It is easy to see that the dog studies for various reasons took place in the water bath under anesthesia. Additionally, there is a differing "density" of pain receptors in skin and tissue which makes it impossible to simply carry over the results of these tests to people. Therefore human application must begin under general anesthesia. By observation of general pain responses, such as blood pressure and pulse rate under various depths of anesthesia, it will be possible to determine to what extent general anesthesia can be eliminated.

It is not theoretically impossible to assume, in fact it is even believed, that this shock wave exposure can be carried out under a very light sedation, and this will of course create a new aspect in the treatment of risk patients where, based on a high internal risk, operative removal of stones is not possible. This not only creates an alternative to the now used surgical stone removal, it could present the only possible form of therapy for these patients.

In about 20 % of the stone patients the first diagnosis states staghorn calculi [66]. Currently, the treatment method most often chosen is complete removal of the concretion to avoid a consequent kidney damage which can lead to kidney insufficiency on both sides. Unfortunately, it is only possible in a few cases to remove all concretions in massive kidney stone disease through a tissue-protective pyelolithotomy. The removal of stones reaching up into the smallest calyces demands a transparenchymal procedure besides renal ischemia. By this, an irreversible disfunction of the parenchyma of the kidney cannot be avoided. *May* [66] found that with such operations there is an average irreversible functional loss of the stone carrying kidney of 20 %.

The pre-operative shock wave exposure of staghorn calculi is a possibility for avoiding such functional losses. But one cannot expect that it will lead to a spontaneous discharge of such a large quantity of stones but it is possible to flush out the individual pieces by irrigation of the collecting system and therefore to avoid a nephrotomy. How far irrigation through a percutaneous, transrenal kidney fistula can be conducted and exposure of the kidney avoided can only be shown through clinical application.

With all these speculative discussions concering clinical application the fact remains that the here described studies show for the first time the proof that in principle a therapeutic use of high energy shock waves in the area of biology and medicine is possible. Naturally, the final adaption to clinical application requires a high investment and further design work based on the conclusions and apparatus outlined in this work, which in the authors' opinion is well worthwhile. On the other hand, it can be assumed that the contact-free destruction of kidney stones will not be the only area of clinical application of shock waves.

# Summary

A method for the contact-free destruction of urinary stones through extracorporeally generated shock waves was developed, and the results were presented in both in vivo and in vitro studies.

The shock waves were produced by a spark gap in the focal region of a water-filled semi-ellipsoid, and, by reflection on the inner wall of the ellipsoid, they converge in the second focal point. The material to be exposed was placed in this focus.

1. In technical pretrials, it was proven that a change and an increase in pressure amplitude of the shock wave could be achieved through widening the distance between the electrodes or through increase in the condenser discharge voltage. There is a correlation between the rate of the discharge of the circuit and the shock wave intensity. Interposition of tissue layers between the first and second focal points of the ellipsoid does not influence the focusing of the shock wave but leads to a damping of the pressure amplitude.

2. In the first in vitro studies urinary stones of different chemical compositions were reproducibly disintegrated when placed in the focal area. Exposure of human erythrocytes and lymphocytes to shock waves with equal energy leads to no appreciable traumatizing which would exclude clinical application. In addition, there was no influence on the proliferative cell mechanism.

   These results were confirmed with a shock wave application to the rat. With the exception of the exposure to the thoracic region which led to alveolar damage, there was no tissue traumatizing, either by specific exposure of individual organs or general exposure of the abdominal region.

3. After development of an experimental stone model, an in vivo urinary stone destruction was achieved by shock wave exposure. It was shown that locating of implanted kidney stones was possible with none of the available ultrasonic systems. But it could be proven that destruction of kidney stones with shock waves brought about pathological changes in neither the area of the kidney nor the surrounding tissue.

4. A reproducible locating of kidney stones was obtainable through integration of a two axis X-ray system. With this and a spark discharge of lower energy in comparison with that of the pretrials the implanted kidney

stones in the dogs were reproducibly disintegrated so that they could be spontaneously discharged, even with this form of application there were no function-influencing defects or systematically provable damage found.

*Acknowledgements*

The authors hereby wish to express sincere thanks for the generous support which they received during the process of these investigations. Our special gratitude is due to Ms. H. Bayer, who worked on this project as chief medical assistant. We would also especially like to thank Dr. W. Wieland and Dr. K. Wanner for their help in our animal experiments. Dr. Rindfleisch, Professor Dr. K. Pielsticker, Dr. E. Moser and Professor Dr. U. Büll for auxiliary experiments in the course of this work.

## Literature

1. *Aboulker, P.; Thomas, J.; Boyer, C.; Momal, J.-P.; Motz, C.; Wetterwald, F.:* Dissolution of phosphate and oxalate calculi. Presse méd. 74, 2843 (1966)
2. *Alken, C. E.; Dix, V. W.; Weyrauch, H. M.; Wildbolz, E.:* Die Steinerkrankungen. Handbuch der Urologie, Bd. X. Springer, New York, Berlin 1961
3. *Anderson, L.; Mc Donald, J. R.:* The origin, frequency and significance of microscopic calculi in the kidney. Surg. Gynec. Obstet. 82, 275 (1946)
4. *Anderson, C. K.:* Partial nephrectomy – a pathological evaluation. Proc. Roy. Soc. Med. 67, 459 (1974)
5. *Badenoch, A. W.:* Uric acid stone formation. Brit. J. Urol. 32, 374 (1960)
6. *Bailitis, E.:* Der Schallimpuls eines Flüssigkeitsfunkens. Z. f. angew. Physik einschl. Nukleonik 9, 429 (1957)
7. *Balzerowiak, H.-P.; Prümmer, R.:* Das elektrohydraulische Umformverfahren in der Praxis. Z. f. wirt. Fort. 67, 246 (1972)
8. *Blacllock, N. J.:* The pattern of urolithiasis in the Royal Navy. In: Renal Stone Research Symposium Eds. Hodgkinson, A., Nordin, B. E. C., London, Churchill, p. 33 (1969)
9. *Blandy, J.:* Urology. Blackwell Scientific Publications, Oxford 1976
10. *Boyce, W. H.; Garvey, F. K.; Strawcutter, H. F.:* Incidence of urinary calculi among patients in general hospitals 1948-1952. J. Amer. med. Ass. 161, 1437 (1956)
11. *Boyce, W. H.; Sulkin, N. M.:* Biocolloids of urine in health and in calculous disease. III. The mucoprotein matrix of urinary calculi. J. Clin. Invest. 35, 1067 (1956)
12. *Boyce, W. H.; Pool, C. S.; Meschan, I.; King, J. S.:* Organic matrix of urinary calculi. Acta Radiol. 50, 544 (1958)
13. *Boyce, W. H.; King, J. S.; Fielden, M. L.:* Total non-dialysable solids in human urine, XIII. Immunological detection of a component peculiar to renal calculous matrix and to urine of calculous patients. J. Clin. Invest. 41, 1180 (1962)
14. *Brendel, W.; Albers, C.; Usinger, W.:* Der Kreislauf in Hypothermie. Pflügers Archiv Ges. Physiol. 266, 357 (1958a)
15. *Buchton, K. E.; Baher, N. V.:* An investigation into possible chromosome damaging effects of ultrasound on human blood cells. Brit. J. Radiol. 45, 340 (1972)
16. *Büttger, B.:* Zur elektrohydraulischen Lithotripsie von Blasensteinen mit Urat I (YPAT-1). Z. Urol. 62, 495 (1969)
17. *Burch, P. R. J.; Dawson, J. B.:* Aetiological implications of the sex- and agedistributions of renal lithiasis. In: Renal Stone Research Symposium. Eds. Hodgkinson, A., Nordin, B. E. C., London, Churchill, p. 71 (1969)
18. *Carr, R. J.:* Aetiology of renal calculi: micro-radiographic-studies. In: Renal Stone Research Symposium. Eds. Hodgkinson, A., Nordin, B. E. C., London, Churchill, p. 123 (1969)
19. *Chaussy, Ch.; Eisenberger, F.; Wanner, K.; Forssmann, B.; Hepp, W.; Schmiedt, E.; Brendel, W.:* The use of shock waves for the destruction of renal calculi without direct contact. Urological Research 4, 175 (1976)
20. *Chaussy, Ch.; Eisenberger, F.; Wanner, K.; Forssmann, B.; Hepp, W.:* In vitro-Untersuchungen und erste in vivo-Untersuchungen mit fokussierten Stoßwellen. Biophysikalische Verfahren zur Diagnose und Therapie von Steinleiden der Harnwege. Wissenschaftliche Berichte, Meersburg Juni (1976)
21. *Chaussy, Ch.; Eisenberger, F.; Wanner, K.:* Die Implantation humaner Nierensteine – ein einfaches experimentelles Steinmodell. Urologe A 16, 35 (1977)
22. *Chaussy, Ch.; Eisenberger, F.; Wanner, K.; Forssmann, B.:* Extracorporale Anwendung von hochenergetischen Stoßwellen. Ein neuer Aspekt in der Behandlung des Harnsteinleidens; Teil II. Aktuelle Urologie 9, 95 (1978)

23 *Chaussy, Ch.; Schmiedt, E.; Forssmann, B.; Brendel, W.:* Contact free renale stone destruction by means of shock waves. Europ. Surg. Res. *11*, 36 (1979)
24 *Coats, C. E.:* The application of ultrasonic energy to urinary and biliary calculi. J. Urol. *75*, 865 (1956)
25 *Council, W. A.:* The treatment of ureteral calculi; report of 504 cases in which Council stone extractor and dilator was used. J. Urol. *53*, 534 (1945)
26 *David, E.:* Physikalische Vorgänge bei elektrischen Drahtexplosionen. Z. F. Physik *150*, 162 (1958)
27 *Eisenberger, F.; Chaussy, Ch.; Wanner, K.:* Entwicklung eines steintragenden Hundemodells zur in vivo-Untersuchung der Wirkung fokussierter Stoßwellen auf Nierensteine. Biophysikalische Verfahren zur Diagnose und Therapie von Steinleiden der Harnwege. Wissenschaftliche Berichte, Meersburg Juni (1976)
28 *Eisenberger, F.; Schmiedt, E.; Chaussy, Ch.; Wanner, K.; Forssmann, B.; Hepp, W.:* Aspekte zum derzeitigen Stand der berührungsfreien Harnsteinzertrümmerung. Deutsches Ärzteblatt *17*, 1145 (1977)
29 *Eisenberger, F.; Chaussy, Ch.; Wanner, K.:* Extracorporale Anwendung von hochenergetischen Stoßwellen – Ein neuer Aspekt in der Behandlung des Harnsteinleidens. Akt. Urol. *8*, 3 (1977)
30 *Fabiano, A.:* Die elektrische Lithotripsie von Steinen der Harnwege unter besonderer Berücksichtigung der transvesicalen Uretersteinzertrümmerung. Endoscopy *2*, 157 (1970)
31 *Fleisch, H.; Bisaz, S.:* Mechanism of calcification: inhibitory role of pyrophosphate. Nature *195*, 911 (1962 b)
32 *Forssmann, B.; Hepp, W.; Chaussy, Ch.; Eisenberger, F.; Wanner, K.:* Zertrümmerung von Nierensteinen mit fokussierten Stoßwellen. Verhandl. DPG (VI) 11, K 4 (1976)
33 *Forssmann, B.; Hepp, W.; Chaussy, Ch.; Eisenberger, F.; Wanner, K.:* Eine Methode zur berührungsfreien Zertrümmerung von Nierensteinen durch Stoßwellen. Biomed. Techn. *22*, 164 (1977)
34 *Forster, D.; Thammen, H.:* Zur Infektionsprophylaxe bei retrograden Untersuchungen der oberen Harnwege. Med. Welt *30*, 932 (1979)
35 *Fox, M.; Pyrak, L. N.; Ruper, F. P.:* Management of ureteric stone: Review of 292 cases. Brit. J. Urol. *37*, 660 (1965)
36 *Gellissen, H.; Reuter, H. J.:* Erste Erfahrungen mit der elektrohydraulischen Lithotripsie von Harnleitersteinen. Z. Urol. *66*, 81 (1974)
37 *Goldman, D. E.; Hueter, T. F.:* Tabular Data of the Velocity and Absorption of High-Frequency Sound in Mammalian Tissues. J. acous. Soc. Amer. *28*, 35 (1956)
38 *Hartung, R.; Egger, B.; Riedhammer, F.:* Die operative Therapie des Nierensteinleidens. Med. Welt *30*, 950 (1979)
39 *Häusler, E.; Kiefer, W.:* Anregung von Stoßwellen in Flüssigkeiten durch Hochgeschwindigkeitswassertropfen. Verhandlungen DPG, Frühjahrstagung in Ulm, K. 36 (1971)
40 *Häusler, E.:* Druckwellen gegen Nierensteine. Amphora Nr. 4 (1975)
41 *Häusler, E.; Kiefer, W.:* Zerstörung von spröden Einschlüssen in flüssiger Umgebung durch autofokussierte Stoßwellen. Verhandl. DPG (VI) 10, K 35 (1975)
42 *Häusler, E.; Kiefer, W.:* Destruction of kidney stones by means of autofocussed guided shockwaves. 2nd European Congress on Ultrasonics in Medicine, München (1975)
43 *Hamman, J.-F.:* Stoß- und Druckwellen und ihre Umformwirkung beim Hydrospark-Verfahren. Z. angew. Physik *31*, 133 (1971)
44 *Heise, G. W.; Müller, G. W.:* Beiträge zur Entstehung und Auflösung von Harnsteinen. Urologe A *4*, 171 (1966)

45 *Hellmann, L. K.; Dufus, G. K.; Donald J.; Sunden, B.:* Safety of diagnostic ultrasound in obstectrics. Lancet I, 113 (1970)
46 *Hellstrom, J.:* Erfahrungen über Entstehung, Wachstum und spontanen Abgang von Nierensteinen. Z. Urol. Chir. *18*, 248 (1925)
47 *Hepp, W.:* Vorversuche zur Zerkleinerung von Nierensteinen durch Stoßwellen. Dornier System, Versuchsbericht 638 (1972)
48 *Hochheimer, B. F.:* Lasers in Ophthalmology. In: Laser Applications in Medicine and Biology. Ed. Wolbarsht, M. L. Plenum Press, New York, London, Vol. 2 (1974)
49 *Howards, S.; Merrill, E.; Harris, S.; Cohen, J.:* Effect of Ultrasonic Irradiation on Urinary calculi and Urothelium. Surgical Forum XXIII (1972)
50 *Hüter, J.:* Messung der Ultraschallabsorption in tierischen Geweben und ihre Abhängigkeit von der Frequenz. Naturwissenschaften *35*, 285 (1948)
51 *Johnson, R. G.; Stiefbold, B. L.:* The effect of urea, magnesium chloride and a low protein diet on the production of calcium oxalate vesical calculi in the rat. J. Urol. (Baltimore) *81*, 691 (1959)
52 *Kawamura, J.; Hosohawa, S.; Yoskida, O.; Fujita, T.; Ischii, Y.; Torizuka, K.:* Validity of $99^m$ Tc Dimercaptosuccinic acid renal uptake for an assessment of individual kidney function. J. Urol. *119*, 305 (1978)
53 *Kern, E.:* Entwicklung einer Sonde zur Zertrümmerung von Uretersteinen durch Elektro-Lithotripsie. Biomed. Technik *18*, 21 (1973)
54 *Keyser, L. D.:* The etiology of urinary lithiasis: an experimental study. Arch. Surg. *6*, 523 (1923)
55 *Kiefhaber, P.:* Endoskopische Blutstillung mit Laserstrahlen. Fortschr. Med. *94*, 656 (1974)
56 *Kiefhaber, P., Teufel, H., Moritz, K.:* Erste Laserendoskopie mit einem flexiblen Transmissionssystem. Fortschritte der Endoskopie, Bd. 6. F. K. Schattauer, Stuttgart, New York (1975)
57 *Kierfeld, G.:* Lithotripsie von Blasensteinen durch hydraulische Schlagwellenwirkung. Verh. Ber. d. dt. Ges. f. Urologie, Berlin (1968)
58 *Kierfeld, G.; Mellin, P.; Daum, H.:* Blasensteinzertrümmerung durch hydraulische Schlagwellenwirkung im Tierexperiment. Urologe *8*, 99 (1969)
59 *Kirk, J. W.:* Impulse Forming by Electrical Discharge Methods. Sheet Metal Industries *39*, 533 (1962)
60 *Kolle, P.:* Der Harnsäurestein. Münchn. med. Wschr. *109*, 245 (1967)
61 *Kollwitz, A. A.:* Auflösung von Harnsäuresteinen durch orale Alkalisierung. Urologe A *3*, 197 (1964)
62 *Lamport, H.; Newmann, H. F.:* Ultrasonic lithotresis in the ureter. J. Urol. *76*, 520 (1955)
63 *Lamport, H.; Newmann, H. F.:* A critical appraisal of methods for disruption and extraction of urinary calculi, especially with ultrasound. Yale J. Biol. and Med. *27*, 395 (1955)
64 *Linke, Ca. A.; Carstensen, E. L.; Frizzel, L. A.; Elbadawi, A.; Fridd, C. W.:* Localized Tissue destruction by high-intensity focused ultrasound. Arch. Surg. *107*, 887 (1973)
65 *Loch, E. G.:* Kritische Betrachtung über mögliche Nebenwirkungen der Ultraschalldiagnostik. Gynäkologe *9*, 103 (1976)
66 *May, P.:* Nierenbeckenausgußsteine – Grenzen der Operabilität. Urologe A *13*, 244 (1974)
67 *Mc Guff, P. E.:* Surgical Application of Laser. Ed. Charles C. Thomas. Springfield USA (1966)
68 *Müller, H.:* Hydroelektrische Umformung, das Umformverfahren mit Hilfe einer Stoßstromanlage. Mitt. Forsch. Ges. Blechverarbeitung Nr. 5/6, 102 (1965)
69 *Mürtz, H.-J.:* Hochspannungs-Explosionsumformung. ETZ-B *19*, 529 (1964)

70 *Ouchi, T.; Takakaski, H.:* Desintegration of urinary calculi by means of ultrasonic vibration. Kong. Int. Ges. Urol. München (1967)
71 *Pyrah, L. N.:* Renal calculus. Springer Verlag Berlin, Heidelberg, New York (1979)
72 *Randall, A.:* The origin and growth of renal calculi. Ann Surg. *105,* 1009 (1937)
73 *Rathert, P.:* Ultraschall in der Behandlung der Urolithiasis. Therapiewoche *26* (1976)
74 *Reuter, H. J.; Kern, E.:* Electronic Lithotripsy of Ureteral Calculi. J. Urol. *110,* 181 (1973)
75 *Rinehart, J. S.:* The Role of Stress Waves in the Comminution of Brittle, Rocklike Materials. Int. Symp. Stress Waves Prop. In Materials New York, 247 (1967)
76 *Rott, H. D.; Soldner, R.; v. ZYL, J.:* Zur Wirkung von Ultraschall auf menschliche Chromosomen in vitro. Geburtsh. u. Frauenheilk., *32,* 662 (1972)
77 *Rosenbach, F.:* Kritische und experimentelle Beiträge zur Frage der Entstehung der Nierensteine. Mitt. a. d. Grenzgeb. d. Med. u. Chir. *12,* 630 (1911)
78 *Sandegard, E.:* Prognosis of stone in the ureter. Acta Chri. Scand., Suppl. 219 (1956)
79 *Sandegard, E.:* The results of expectant treatment of urolithiasis: follow up study of kidney function and recurrence. Acta Chir. Scand. *116,* 44 (1958)
80 *Schade, H.:* Beiträge zur Konkrementbildung. Zur Entstehung der Harnsteine. Münch. med. Wschr. *56,* 77 (1909)
81 *Schall, R.:* Detonationsphysik. In: Kurzzeitphysik, Vollrath, K., Thomer, G. (Ed.) Springer Verlag, Wien (1967)
82 *Schmiedt, E.:* Diagnostik des Harnsteinleidens. Biophysikalische Verfahren zur Diagnose und Therapie von Steinleiden der Harnwege. Meersburg (1976)
83 *Schuy, S.; Schmidt-Kloiber, H.:* Methoden zur Zerstörung von Nieren-, Harnleiter- und Blasensteinen. Biomedizinische Technik *18,* 17 (1973)
84 *Staehler, W.:* Klinik und Praxis der Urologie. Thieme, Stuttgart (1959)
85 *Staehler, G.:* Zerstörung von Blasentumoren durch endoskopische Applikation von Laserstrahlen. Habilitationsschrift, München (1977)
86 *Steward, H. H.:* Calcification and calculous formation in the upper urinary tract. Brit. J. Urol. *27,* 352 (1953)
87 *Sutherland, J. W.:* Recurrence following operations for upper urinary tract stone. Brit. J. Urol. *26,* 22 (1954)
88 *Terhorst, B.; Cichos, M.:* Ultraschall zur Harnsteinzertrümmerung (Experimentelle Untersuchungen). Biomed. Technik *16,* 106 (1971)
89 *Terhorst, B.; Lutzeyer, W.; Cichos, M.; Pohlmann, R.:* Die Zerstörung von Harnsteinen durch Ultraschall. II. Ultraschall-Lithotripsie von Blasensteinen. Urol. int. *27,* 458 (1972)
90 *Terhorst, B.; Cichos, M.:* Ultraschall zur Harnsteinzertrümmerung (Klinische Ergebnisse). Biomed. Technik *18,* 13 (1973)
91 *Terhorst, B.:* Blasensteinbehandlung durch Ultraschall. Dtsch. Ärzteblatt *71,* 519 (1974)
92 *Terhorst, B.; Cichos, M.; Versin, F.; Bus, H.:* Der Einfluß von elektrohydraulischen Schlagwellen und Ultraschall auf das Urothel. Urologe A *14,* 41 (1975)
93 *Thomas, W. C.; Howard, J. E.:* Studies on the mineralising propensity of urine from patients with and without calculi. Tans-Ess. Amer. Phys. *72*
94 *Timmermann, A.; Kallistratos:* Modern aspects of chemical dissolution of human renal calculi by irrigation. J. Urol. *95,* 469 (1966)
95 *Verschüren, R.; Odlhoff, J.:* Laser Surgery on Polyps and Tumors of the Rectosigmoid Colon. In: Laser Surgery, Ed.: Kaplan, I., Jerusalem Acad. Press, Jerusalem (1976)
96 *Wanner, K.; Chaussy, Ch.; Eisenberger, F.; Forssmann, B.; Hepp, W.:* Problematik einer integrierten Ultraschallortung im Versuchsmodell „Berührungsfreie Nierenstein-

zertrümmerung". Biophysikalische Verfahren zur Diagnose und Therapie von Steinleiden der Harnwege. Wissenschaftliche Berichte, Meersburg Juni (1976)

97 *Wax, S. H.; Frank, I. N.:* A retrospective study of the upper urinary tract calculi. J. Urol. *94,* 28 (1965)

98 *Williams, R. E.:* Long term survey of 538 patients with upper urinary tract stone. Brit. J. Urol. *35,* 416 (1963)

99 *Williams, R. E.:* The results of conservative surgery for stone. Brit. J. Urol. *44,* 292 (1972)

# 5. Clinical experience with extracorporeal shockwave lithotripsy (ESWL)

## 5.1 History of the clinical application of ESWL

Following the successful and encouraging results accomplished during the 8 years of basic and experimental research (see part 1), an apparatus for clinical use in humans was constructed. The major features of this machine are similar to those of the prototype which was used for the animal experiments: the water tub with the integrated ellipsoid, the biplane X-ray system, the patient support and the control panel (figures 57, 60, 61).

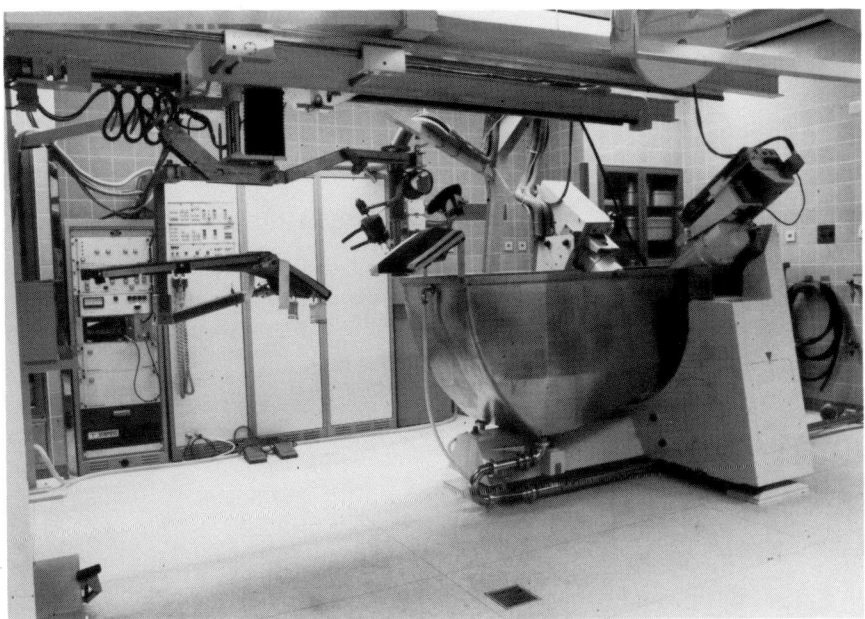

*Figure 57.* Dornier kidney lithotripter. Human model #1.

First human applications started in February of 1980, by *Christian Chaussy* from the Department of Urology of the University of Munich. With this device, the Human Model #1, more than 200 selected patients with kidney stones were treated successfully at the Institute for Surgical Research of the University of Munich [3-5]. In May of 1982, the initial device was replaced by a new revised lithotripter, Human Model #2 (figure 58).

At that time the first lithotripter center consisting of a lithotripter treatment room, adjacent rooms for induction of anesthesia, pre- and post-ESWL X-ray diagnosis, facilities for stone manipulation under fluoroscopy, and offices was opened at the Department of Urology at Munich University, Klinikum Grosshadern. By October of 1983, a third generation device with further improvements, Human Model #3 (figure 59), was available. Between the first clinical use of a lithotripter in 1980, and the second installation in Stuttgart (West

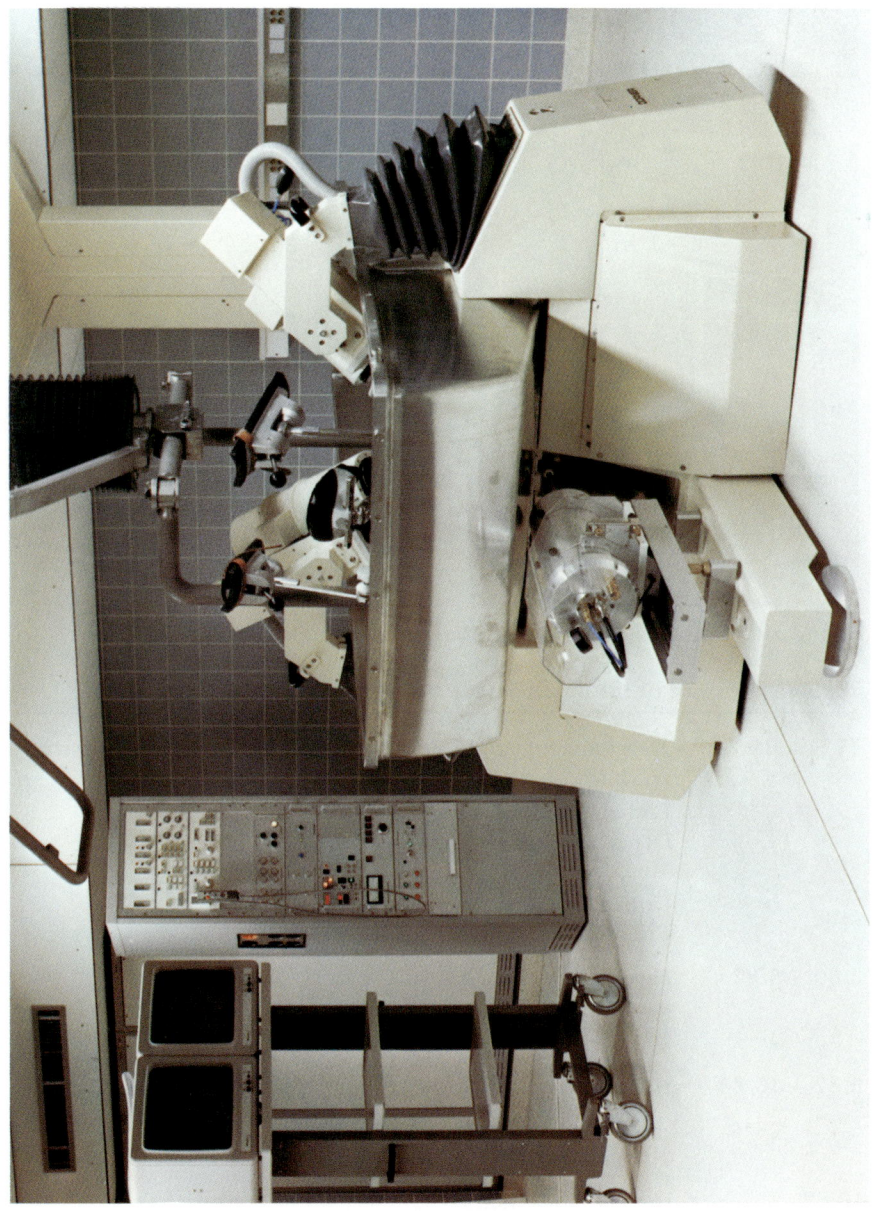

*Figure 58.* Dornier kidney lithotripter. Human model #2.

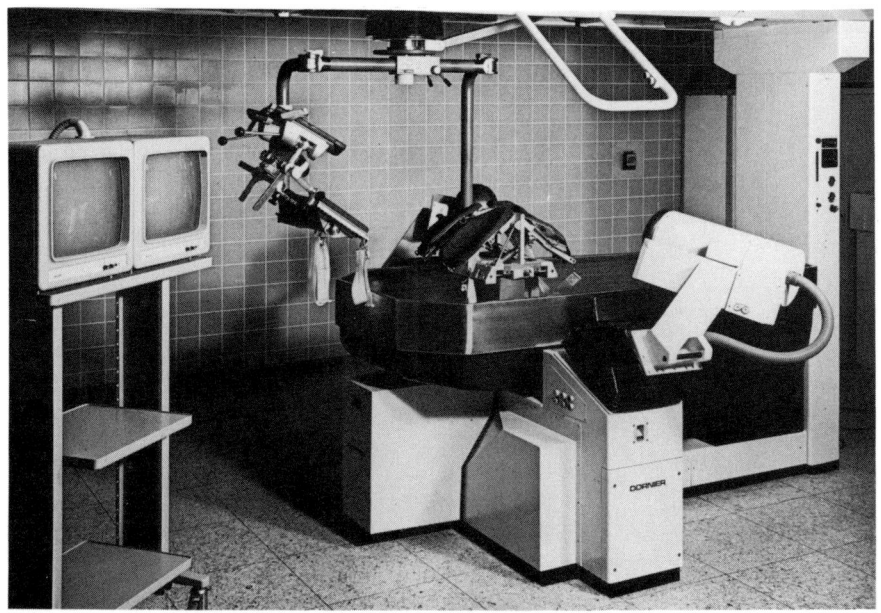

*Figure 59.* Dornier kidney lithotripter. Human model # 3.

*Table IX.* History of the development and distribution of FSWL

| | |
|---|---|
| 1974 – 1980 | *Development of extracorporeal shock wave lithotripsy (ESWL)* |
| | Ludwig Maximilians University<br>Department of Urology<br>Munich, FRG |
| | Dornier Medical Systems<br>Friedrichshafen, FRG |
| 2/80 – 5/82 | *Human model no. 1* |
| | First clinical application of ESWL (Munich, FRG)<br>200 patients |
| 5/82 – 10/83 | *Human model no. 2* |
| | (Munich, FRG)<br>800 patients |
| 10/83 | *Human model no. 3* |
| | Begin series of production and distribution of the lithotripter (Stuttgart, Wuppertal, Berlin, Mainz) |
| 1984 – present | Distribution to 170 centers in 20 countries worldwide |

Germany) by October of 1983, two refined models were constructed based on the Munich experience with more than one thousand patients [5, 6].

This third generation device was the first commercially available lithotripter, and beginning in 1984 it was distributed worldwide (table IX).

## 5.2 Indications for ESWL

### 5.2.1 Patient selection

Based on the experience gained from the animal experiments, which are extensively described in section 1 of this book, it was forseeable that the treatment of humans would also be safe and reliable.

However, as with every method being introduced into clinical use, the initial indications were restricted to get parameter-free conditions and comparable results [2, 3].

The initial exclusion criteria were the following:

1. multiple stones and stones $> 1$ cm,
2. urinary tract infection at the time of treatment,
3. radiolucent stones or semi-opaque stones,
4. risk patients suffering from internal diseases,
5. obstruction distal to the stone, and functional alterations of the upper urinary tract.

The initial indications were confined to patients in good general health presenting with single pelvic stones $< 1$ cm, and single caliceal stones. The size of the stones accepted at first was limited to 1 cm because of the unknown transport capacity of the upper urinary tract for the disintegrated fragments. Further selection criteria were:
anatomical and functional integrity of the upper urinary system to exclude the effect of obstruction, and/or functional alterations on stone discharge.

Presence of a urinary tract infection excluded from ESW-treatment because of the increased possibility of post-ESWL obstructive pyelonephritis. A further prerequisite for eligibility for ESWL was radio-opacity of the stone, as precise radiological localization of the stone deemed mandatory for proper treatment success [2, 3].

This confined the range of patients eligible for ESWL to approx. 20 % of a non-selected patient population. The high success rate achieved with ESWL in this group of selected patients, and the absence of severe complications soon allowed the range of patients eligible for this procedure to be cautiously expanded [2-5].

*Table X.* Present range of ESWL-indications

---
ESWL — indications include:

---
— Single and multiple stones in the kidney and the ureter

— Partial — and complete staghorn stones

— Infected stones

— Stones in solitary kidneys

— High risk patients

— Children ($>$ 120 cm)

— Radiolucent stones

---

Currently, more than 70 % of the nonselected patients are candidates for ESWL as the sole treatment modality, and in combination with endourological methods an additional 20 % — 25 % of the more complicated stone cases become eligible for ESWL, thus reducing the need for open surgery to less than 10 % of all stone patients (table X) [6, 12, 14, 21].

*5.2.2 Current contraindications*

Patients with untreated or untreatable bleeding disorders, and patients with decompensated heart insufficiency are still excluded from treatment with the lithotripter. Technical problems in positioning the patient on the support, and/or localization of the stone into the second focal point exist in grossly obese patients ($>$ 250 lbs.). The upper limit for the patient support is 300 lbs. Patients taller than 6'6", and children smaller than 4'2" can not be positioned on the patient support of the current lithotripter (table XI) [9, 12]. To overcome this shortcoming, which precludes ESWL treatment in approximately 1 % of all stone patients, a new patient support is under construction.

Anatomical alterations of the upper urinary tract can be urological contraindications when strongly influencing the drainage of disintegrated stone material from the kidney. Irregular urodynamic patterns with functional impairment of the motility of the ureter need careful evaluations as to whether or not they preclude successful stone elimination [3, 5, 6, 9-12, 23]. Pregnancy is a firm contraindication for shock wave treatment. The majority of stone cases in pregnancy can be treated conservatively with analgesics and antibiotics. In the rare case where interventional stone treatment has to be considered (unmanageable pain with frequent episodes, imminent urosepsis) placement of a nephrostomy tube under local anesthesia is preferable and suffices in most patients. ESWL can be performed as soon as 14 days post-partum [9].

*Table XI.* Current contraindications

| | |
|---|---|
| *General:* | untreated bleeding disorder<br>not fit for anesthesia<br>pregnancy |
| *Technical:* | gross obesity ($>$ 130 kg)<br>children ($<$ 120 cm)<br>patients $>$ 200 cm |
| *Urologic:* | obstruction distal to the stone<br>caliceal neck stenosis<br>UPJ-stenosis<br>ureteral stenosis<br>BPH; requiring treatment |

## 5.3 Course of the routine ESWL treatment

### 5.3.1 Patient preparation

The indication for ESWL is established the same way as for open surgery (table XII), and the preparations for ESWL are the same as for any conventional surgical stone removal (table XIII). But, there is no need to cross-match blood as the blood loss from the ESW-procedure is negligible [3, 9, 11, 12, 23].

Although, in a small minority of centers, ESWL is being performed in an outpatient setting with little or no special preparation of the patient. Our experience over the years has shown that careful patient preparation secures the quality of the treatment and prevents possible hazards [3-5, 8, 9, 11, 12, 23]. Fluids (1,000-1,500 ml balanced salt solution) administered intravenously beginning the evening before treatment, and continued through the procedure have been found to minimize hypotensive reactions due to the regional anesthesia as well as side effects of the shock waves on the renal parenchyma [9]. No further measures are necessary before ESWL aside from the administration of carminatives, which are administered the day before treatment in order to have the bowels free of air on the day of treatment to ensure good X-ray visualization of the targeted stone(s).

*Table XII.* Evaluation of the ESWL-patient

1. History and physical examination
2. Intravenous pyelogram (IVP), not older than 3 months, or if patient is allergic plain abdominal X-ray and retrograde pyelogram
3. Urinalysis and urine culture
4. Optional: split renal function and nephrotomograms

*Table XIII.* Course of the routine ESWL-procedure

A. *Day of admission*

  1. Chest X-ray, EKG
  2. Laboratory data: Hbg., Hkt., leukocytes, creatinine, BUN, clotting profile (PT, PTT, platelets, bleeding time), urinalysis and urine culture
  3. Basic examination
  4. Basic examination by anesthesiology and patient consenting for anesthesia
  5. Basic examination by urologist and patient consenting for the procedure
  6. Installation of I.V. line (1,000 – 1,500 ccs. of balanced sodium solution prior to ESWL and antibiotics, if needed)

B. *Day of treatment*

  1. Patient stays N.P.O, I.V. infusions are continued and antibiotic administered, if needed (see 5.4.4)
  2. Plain X-ray and ultrasound prior to ESWL
  3. Induction of anesthesia (after KUB of the day has been read by urologist in charge)
  4. ESWL treatment (see 5.4.2, 5.4.3)
     optional: pre-ESWL stent placement in radiolucent stones
     pre-ESWL stone manipulation (in ureteral stones with stents or ureteroscope)
     (in staghorn stones percutaneous debulking as first session)
  5. After ESWL; plain ESWL: plain X-ray and ultrasound
  6. Recovery room

C. *After care*

  1. On return to the ward: IV discontinued, patient mobilized, and fluid intake of 2-3 l/day
  2. Examinations: ultrasound to exclude side effects, KUB and ultrasound to assess degree of stone disintegration and monitor stone passage

*Table XIII.*  Continuation

D. *Follow-up*

1. High fluid intake continued, physical activity
2. Examinations:
   - 2 weeks follow-up: KUB
     optional: ultrasound
   - if stone free at 2 weeks, 3 months follow-up:
     KUB, ultrasound, urinalysis, urine culture, blood pressure
   - if not stone free at 2 weeks, additional check ups in 2 – 4 weeks intervals

On the day of treatment before induction of anesthesia, a plain X-ray (KUB) is obtained to verify the exact position of the stone, and to exclude strong shadowing by intestinal gas. Both, experimental studies and clinical experience have shown that shock wave treatment in the presence of intestinal gas does not cause any traumatization of the region involved. However, localization of small stones and assessment of the degree of stone disintegration is more difficult. Therefore, in cases with extreme shadowing due to overlying air treatment is postponed (table XIII) [6, 7, 11].

*5.3.2 Anesthesia*

Anesthesia is mandatory as shock wave therapy is otherwise painful. Although the pain caused by individual shock waves could be tolerated, studies with volunteers have shown that the pain caused by a series of shock waves as it would be in a treatment, can not be tolerated.
In almost all centers, epidural catheter anesthesia has been the method of choice. At those centers, this kind of anesthesia is being used in 75 % – 95 % of all patients.

The indwelling epidural catheter offers the possibility of easily stepping up the anesthesia should the procedure be delayed (staged procedure), or prolonged (combination therapy in ureteral and radiolucent stones). To prevent catheter related infection the catheter entry site is sealed water-tight with a surgical incision drape, and checked by the anesthesiologist on a daily basis [8, 9, 12, 14, 23].

At those centers where regional anesthesia is the preferred mode of anesthesia, general anesthesia is only performed if there are contraindications for regional anesthesia, or if requested by the patient. In high risk patients, general anesthesia is preferred as it permits more extensive monitoring (CVP, PWP, AP), and in children to prevent uncontrolled movement during the procedure and keep breath excursions shallow.

It should be mentioned that a few centers favor the sole use of general anesthesia. The arguments for this are the higher patient turnover, and the fact that most anesthesiologists are not as well trained in performing epidural anesthesia [8, 14].

Attempts at using local anesthetics with sedation and the use of Ketamine anesthesia are limited to very few centers. The local anesthetics are injected subcutaneously to the skin entry site of the shock waves and the lower ribs. Preliminary results indicate that both methods seem to be applicable to only a few patients, and the results have not been confirmed yet in larger series [8, 14].

### 5.3.3 Shock wave treatment

After induction of the appropriate anesthesia, the patient is brought to the lithotripter room where he is placed on the patient support. The patient is fixed on the support with straps to prevent involuntary movement during the treatment due to buoyancy once he is immersed in the water (figure 60).

The patient support is then manually moved over the tub and the patient immersed in the water. After the patient is suspended in the water bath, the stones are localized using the biplane X-ray system. Once the stone is moved in a way that it is in the center of the hairpins on both monitors, it is exactly located on the focal area of the shock wave front and treatment commences (figure 61).

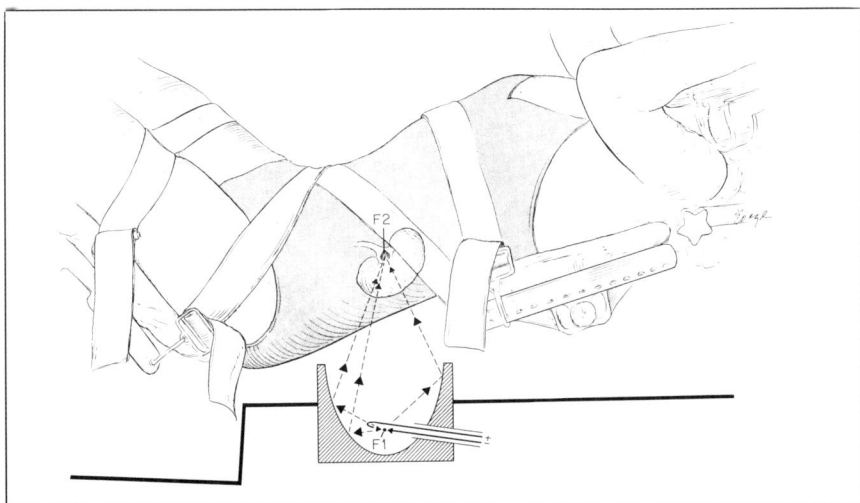

*Figure 60.* Patient on patient support with schematic drawing of the ellipsoid with spark gap (F1) and stone in focal area F2.

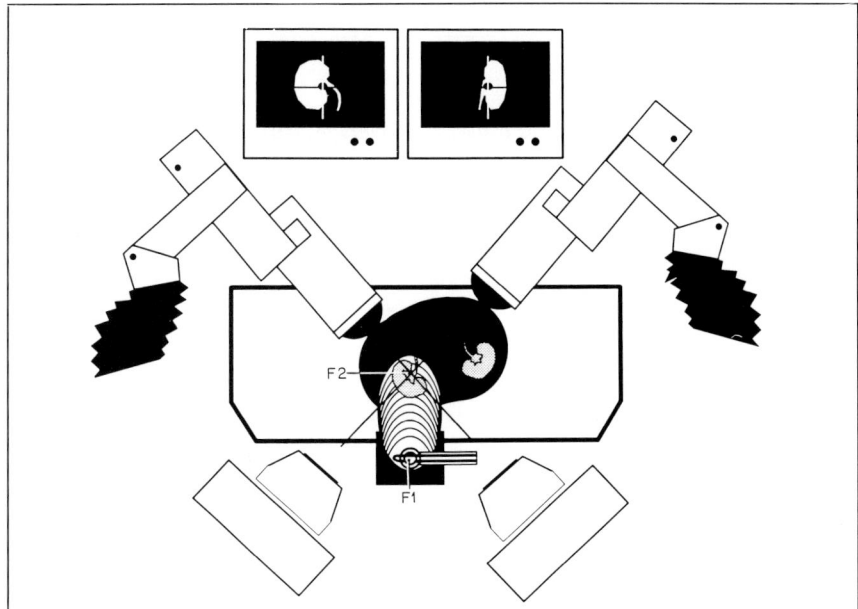

*Figure 61.* Schematic drawing of X-ray localization system, ellipsoid with spark gap in F1, stone centered in F2.

After every 100 shock wave exposures, fluoroscopy is employed and/or frame pictures are taken to assess the degree of stone disintegration. During treatment the stone(s) are repositioned as necessary using fluorscopy until complete disintegration of all stone parts is achieved [2-9, 11, 23].

a) ECG triggering of the shock wave

The individual shock wave is triggered 170 msec. after the steep onset of the R-wave of the ECG. This insures that the shock wave is being delivered during the repolarization phase of the heart cycle, and therefore does not initiate extrasystoles as it does not interfere with the proper conduction. Employing this R-wave, linked triggering has sharply reduced the incidence of ESW-induced extrasystoles. Extrasystoles which were rather frequently encountered among the first patients are now seen in less than 1 % of patients. Even pre-existing severe cardiac arrhythmia does not necessarily preclude ESWL. Within a heart rate range of 40 — 100/min, no major negative side effects have been observed. In cases of tachycardia, or tachyarrhythmia with a frequency greater 100/min, the unit offers the option to omit every other trigger point. This way the minimal shock wave capacitor loading time of 0.47 sec can be obeyed, and treatment conducted as usual. When the frequency is higher than 120/min, ESWL is discontinued and medical therapy instituted. In most cases, ESWL can be resumed after the heart rate is back to normal and the cardiocirculatory

*Table XIV.* Treatment data

| | |
|---|---|
| # of shock waves (500 – 2,000) | average: 1,350 |
| Duration of treatment (20 – 60 min) | average: 45 min |
| *Radiation* | |
| Fluoroscopy time (100 ± 80 sec) | average: 105 sec |
| Frame pictures | average: 8 – 14 |

parameters are stable. Treatment has very rarely been terminated ($<$ 0.5 %) owing to cardiovascular complications [9, 12, 14, 23].

b) Treatment data

Depending upon the stone size, hardness, and number of stones, the individual treatment consists of 500 – 2,000 repeated shock wave applications and lasts for 20 – 60 min (table XIV).
X-ray exposure of the patient due to fluoroscopy (100 ± 80 sec) and the frame pictures (8-14) is in the range of 3-5 rads. This is similar to the radiation incurred during one IVP examination consisting of 3-5 X-ray films [3-9, 11, 12, 23].

c) Side effects

During shock wave treatment slight macrohematuria is detected in all patients. This is attributed to small lesions of the mucoid lining where disintegrated stone material is in direct contact with the wall of the collecting system. The hematuria usually subsides within a few hours. The amount of blood loss is far less than that encountered with any other stone procedure, and is far too small to be picked up by the routinely checked RBC [3, 9, 11, 12, 23].
When the first signs of hematuria are noted during treatment, a 5 mg. dose of lasix is given intravenously to increase the urine output and dilute the urine during the period of the bleeding. With this it is ensured that no clotting in the renal collecting system occurs which eventually might trap stone fragments in narrow segments of the kidney and thus negatively influence proper discharge. Prerequisite for this is a positive pre-ESWL fluid balance which is necessary to make up for the added hypotensive effects of the anesthesia, the warm water and the diuretic agent.
Local symptoms in the area of shock wave entry and exit are observed in a few skinny people. Mainly in very skinny female patients petechiae are noted at the entry site and to a lesser amount at the exit site of the shock wave. The patients have no symptoms whatever and the skin lesions are spontaneously

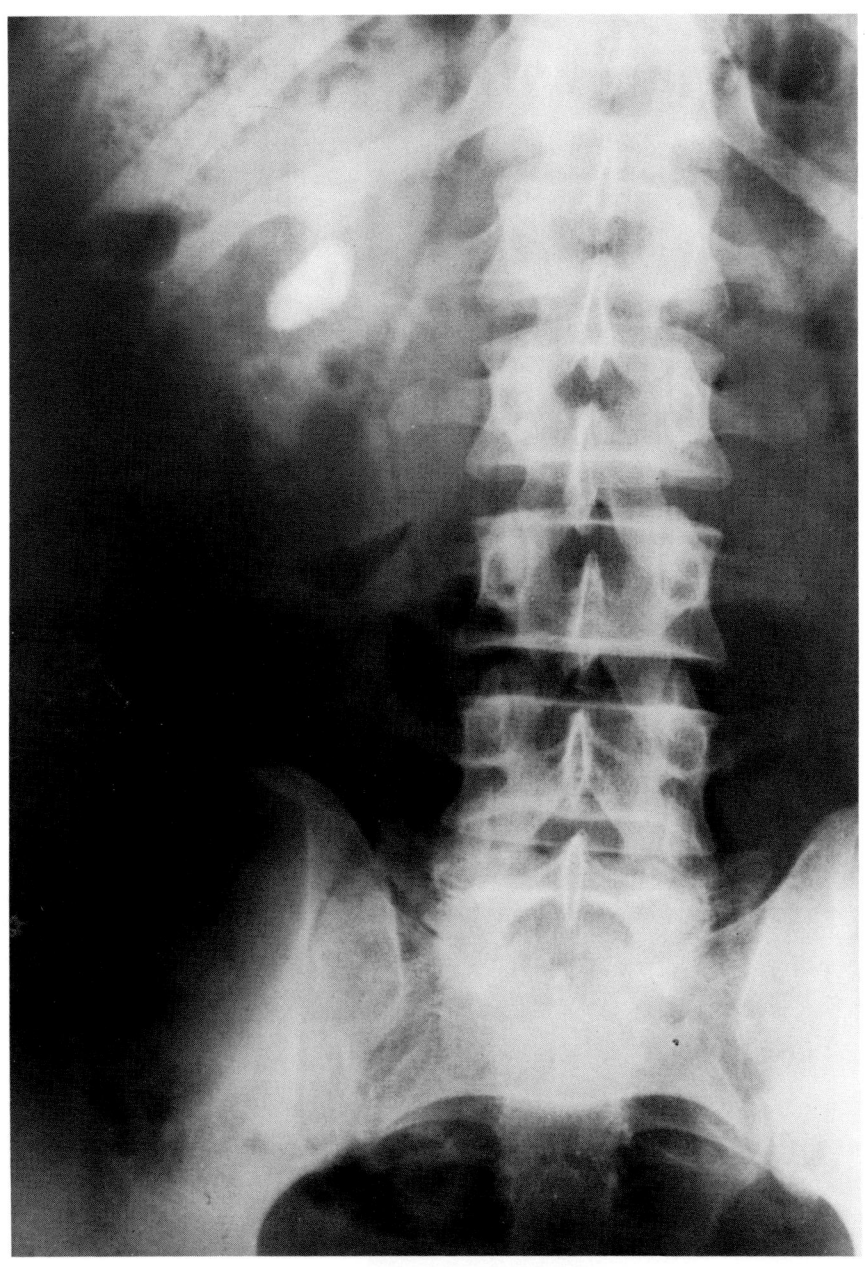

*Figure 62.* Case 1: X-ray control of the ESWL of a renal pelvis stone on the right side
a)  survey radiograph prior to treatment,

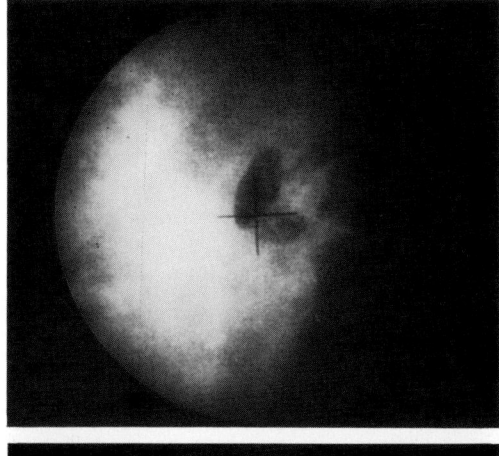

b) after 150,

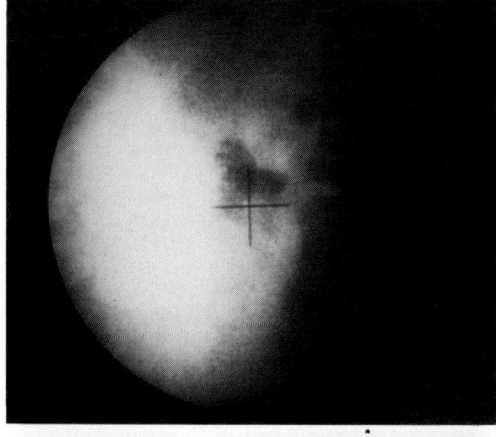

c) after 400,

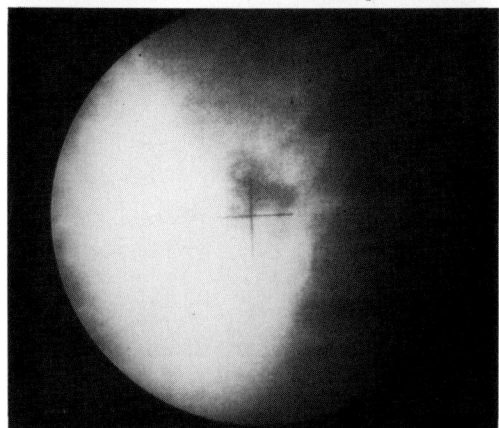

d) after 600 individual shocks,

b-d) monitor images during shock wave treatment

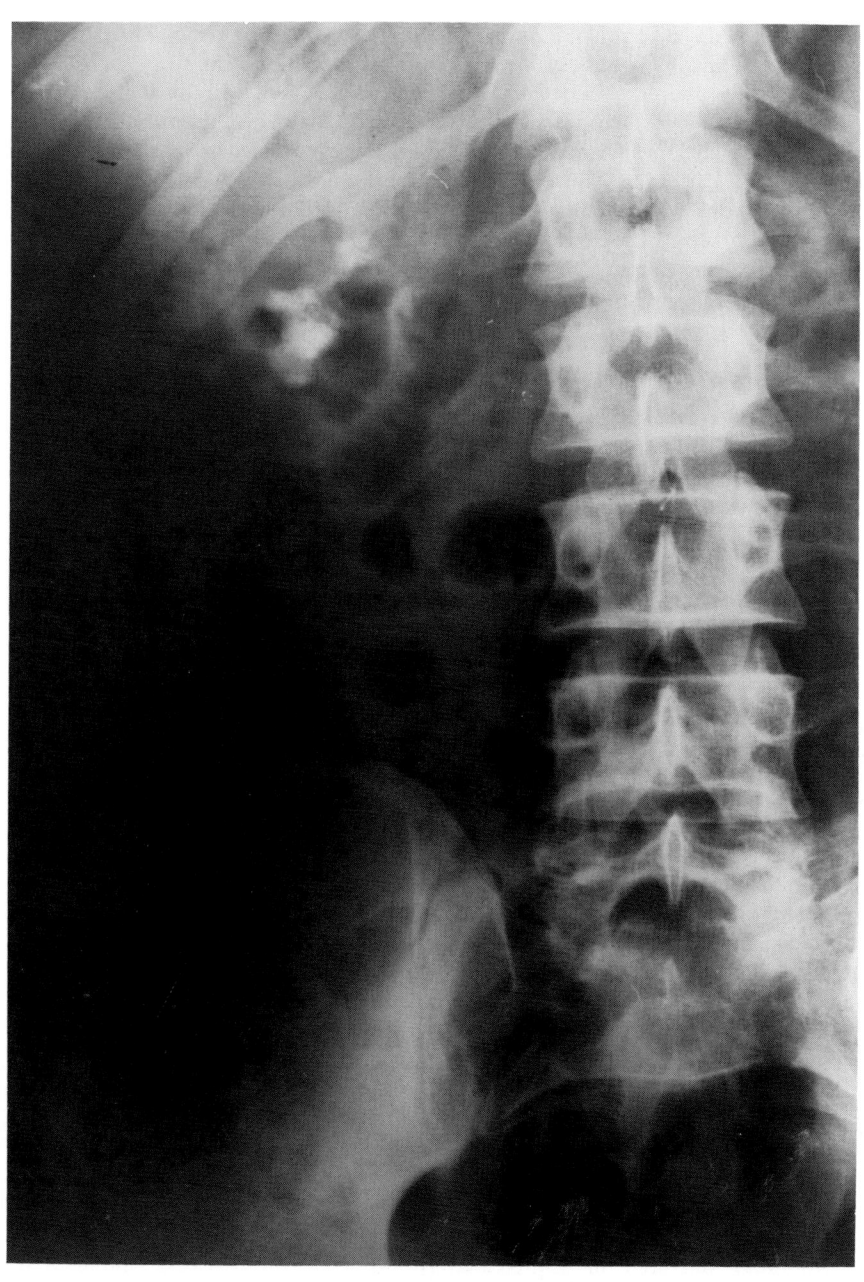

e) final survey radiograph (after 650 individual shocks).

resolved within a couple of days. No correlation between the skin petechiae and any lesions of the kidneys or adjacent organs was ever found.

Those skinny people also occasionally complain of dull pain during the procedure which they localize into the epigastrium. This pain does not change with the level of anesthesia and tends to be more pronounced towards the end of the electrodes' lifespan. Thus, in those patients we usually change the electrodes after 500 shock waves to minimize discomfort. After the treatment, the follow-up of the latter group of patients is similar to that of the normal patient. Most of the aforementioned side effects are irrelevant. The incidence of the skin side effects is in the range of 1 % — 1.5 % of all patients [8, 9, 14].

### 5.3.4  After-care and follow-up

After ESWL treatment is terminated, and the patient removed from the tub, a KUB film is taken to finally assess the degree of stone disintegration (table XIII). If at this time larger fragments are detected, and the upper limit of shock wave application has not been reached (2,000 shock waves per treatment), treatment can be immediately continued as the patient is still under anesthesia. Whenever the KUB shows complete stone disintegration, or a second session is planned, the patient is brought to the recovery room, and after the wear-off of the anesthesia, back to the ward.

There the patient is immediately mobilized, and asked to move as much as possible. The IV line is discontinued as soon as the patient is ambulatory, and the patient is then asked to have a daily oral fluid intake of 2-3 l to maintain a forced diuresis. A basic pain medication is not given, patients get pain medication on request only [3, 9, 11, 23].

The overall experience is that approximately 70 — 90 % of the patients ask for some kind of pain medication during the first 24 h after treatment due to discomfort in the treated area, or at the entry site of the epidural catheter. The incidence of pain or colic related to the treatment itself is relatively low, and varies between 20 and 30 %. Fifty percent of these patients can get relief by oral pain medication, or the use of suppositories. More severe pain attacks, as seen in approximately 10 % of all cases, necessitate IV application of narcotics and reinstitution of intravenous infusions [3, 9, 11, 12, 23].

During the hospital stay, KUB films after treatment are being taken on a daily basis to assess the degree of stone disintegration, and to locate the passing debris. Additional ultrasound examinations are optional. Ultrasound has been proven to be of value as a screening examination for the detection of perirenal fluid collections. In our experience, ultrasound is frequently used during the follow-up. On post-day 1, an ultrasound examination is performed to rule out renal damage and perirenal fluid collections. Thereafter ultrasound is performed to monitor the degree of hydronephrosis, which is to some degree temporarily detected in approximately 60 % of the patients (table XIII) [11, 12].

The rate of patients who leave the hospital stone free depends on the size and location of the original stone(s) and the different policies of hospitalization. In principle, patients are discharged once the KUB confirms complete stone disintegration, and the beginning of the passage of stone fragments. Coincidentally, the ultrasound examination should reveal no perirenal hematoma or evidence of gross hydronephrosis. Ninety percent of the patients can resume their regular work or activities immediately after discharge, and the average disability post-ESWL treatment is 3.5 days (U.S. data).

The out-patient follow-up of the asymptomatic patient consists of a post-day 14 examination (KUB, ultrasound, blood pressure, urinalysis), and at that time further follow-up intervals are determined. If the patient is stone free at this first follow-up visit, or there is only a very small amount of fragments left, then he will be asked back in three months for a follow-up examination including the same procedures (table XIII) [3, 9, 11, 12, 23].

If, at the time of the first follow-up consultation, a moderate amount of fragments remains, and/or the patient reveals a hydronephrosis on ultrasound, then 14 day follow-up intervals are obeyed until the majority of fragments ($> 75\%$) have passed.

This regimen is recommendable, as experience has shown that the severity of post-ESWL complications (obstructive pyelonephritis, urosepsis) is related to patient compliance and follow-up intervals. Thus, close surveillance of those patients who are at risk to sustain post-ESWL complications can not only alleviate the severity of post-ESWL complications, but also results in less invasive auxiliary procedures (endourological procedures versus open surgery or loss of organ) [9].

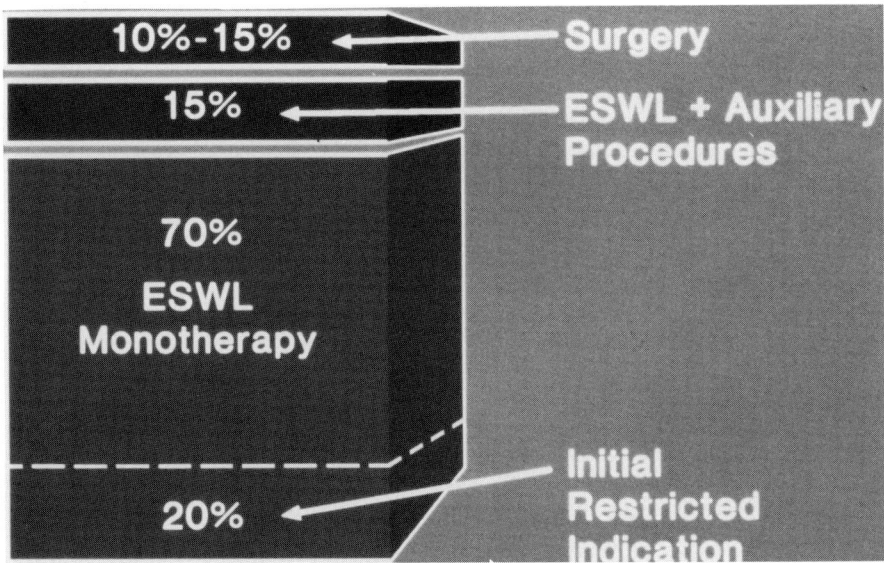

*Figure 63.* Range of ESWL indications; treatment-strategy trends

## 5.4 ESWL management of urinary stones

As mentioned before, most urinary stones are now amenable to ESWL treatment (see 5.2.1; figure 63).
The success of ESWL treatment, a low complication rate and the excellent compliance of patients and involved medical professionals allowed the expansion of the range of indications. The early Munich experience with cautious expansion of patient eligibility finally resulted in the establishment of clearly defined differential indications [3-14, 18, 21, 23]. In the following the current state of ESWL therapy will be described, as well as various combined treatment concepts of ESWL and endourology, and the remaining indications for open surgery will be outlined.

### 5.4.1 Treatment of pelvic and caliceal stones < 2.5 cm

Experience has shown that approximately 70 % of kidney stones can be treated by ESWL monotherapy.

In all kidney stones the rate of successful stone disintegration is in the range of 97 % − 99 %. Only a small minority of all renal stones, namely cystine stones can not be completely reduced in size and require auxiliary procedures. It can by no means be predicted, however, which of these stones will not respond sufficiently [8, 9, 12, 14].
Experience has shown that patients with solitary, or multiple radio-opaque kidney stones of an overall size of up to 2.5 cm, without obstruction distal to the stone can be considered ideal candidates for ESWL treatment with regard to the simplicity of treatment, a high success rate, and a low rate of postprocedural complications [9, 10, 12, 14].
Contrary to other treatment modalities, ESWL offers the advantage that all radiopositive renal stones irrespective of their actual location in the collecting system can be easily localized and treated [1, 3, 11, 17, 19, 24, 25].

### 5.4.2 Treatment of staghorn stones

With increasing experience different strategies have evolved in the treatment of large stones such as partial and complete staghorn stones [3, 5, 7-9, 12, 14, 23].

a) Treatment of staghorn stones filling a nondilated renal collecting system (RCS)

Due to the large overall stone deposit success with one ESWL treatment is the exception. This approach is only feasible in staghorn calculi in nondilated collecting systems (figure 64).

As shown in figure 64a, ESW-treatment of staghorn stones starts at the ureteropelvic junction and there approximately 600-800 shock waves are delivered.

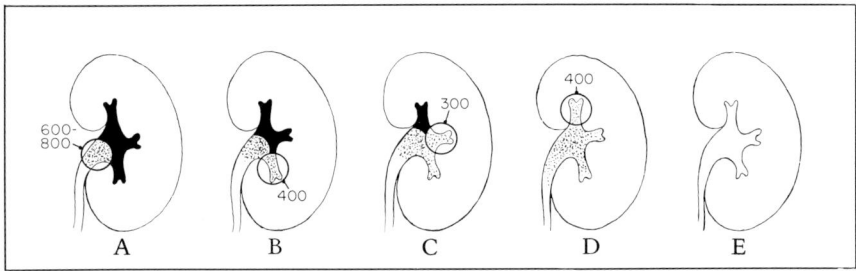

*Figure 64.* Schematic drawing; technique of ESWL treatment of staghorn stones filling a nondilated renal collecting system (RCS).

After this, approximately 400 shock waves are delivered to the lower caliceal group (figure 64b)
Treating the pelvic and the lower caliceal stone parts first eventually facilitates the placement of a percutaneous nephrostomy tube through a lower posterior calyx when required.

The same holds true when the stone does not respond easily and a consecutive treatment has to be undertaken, and between the sessions a percutaneous urinary diversion is needed.

The next step in the routine treatment of a staghorn in a nondilated system is then treatment of the mid caliceal group, where 300 shock waves are spent and then 400 shock waves are applied to the upper calices (figures 64c, d).

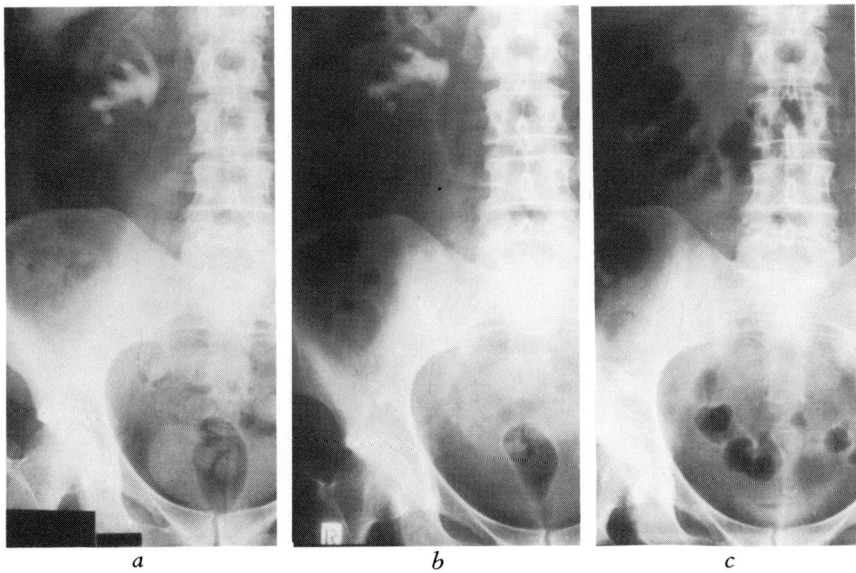

*Figure 65 a-c.* Case 2: ESWL of staghorn stone in a nondilated RCS.

At this point between 1,700-1,900 shock waves have been spent which still leaves a margin of 300-500 shock waves for additional treatment of areas where the stone appears to be not sufficiently fragmented.

Case 2 depicts the treatment course of a typical case of a staghorn stone in a nondilated RCS, treated with an ESWL one-stage procedure.

*Case 2:* 42 years old, male, 1st stone incident, no previous surgery, history of recurrent UTI, current stone analysis: struvite.

Figure 65a shows a complete staghorn stone in a regularly shaped RCS. The stone density is equal to rib densitiy.

One session of ESWL was performed and 1,500 shock waves delivered to the entire stone.

Figure 65b demonstrates complete stone disintegration.

After 6 weeks and an unremarkable follow-up this patient was completely stone free (figure 65c).

b) Treatment of staghorn stones filling mildly dilated RCS

Cases of staghorns with substantially larger stone mass, i.e. when they are filling a larger or a mildly dilated collecting system (equal or larger than hydronephrosis grade I), can be managed in a two stage ESWL procedure which is usually performed within 2-4 days (figure 66).

As shown in figure 66, ESW-treatment of staghorn stones in a slightly dilated RCS starts also at the ureteropelvic junction, and there approximately 800 shock waves are delivered (figure 66b). After this, approximately 600 shock

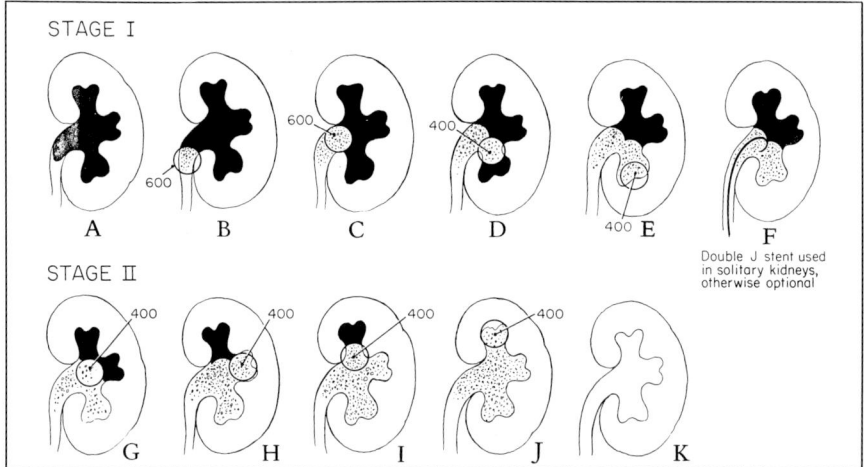

*Figure 66.* Schematic drawing; technique of staged ESWL treatment of staghorn stones filling a slightly dilated RCS.

waves are delivered to the infundibula to the lower caliceal group (figure 66c). Then one of two portions of 400 shock waves each are delivered to the lower calices (figures 66d, e). At this point the first session is terminated with all stone fragments in the renal pelvis and the lower caliceal group disintegrated (figure 66f). If the stone does not respond easily, and larger chunks remain in the treated area, a double-J stent is inserted and left indwelling between the consecutive sessions to prevent larger chunks from falling into the ureter which would necessitate a ureteral manipulation before the following session. This is especially obeyed in staghorn stones in solitary kidneys.

Usually two days after the initial treatment, a second session is undertaken. The next step in the routine treatment is then treatment of the mid caliceal group, where 600-800 shock waves are spent (figure 66g, h). Then 400 shock waves are applied to the upper caliceal infundibula (figure 66i). One to two portions of 400 shock waves each are then delivered to the upper calices (figures 66i, j).

At this point between 1600-2000 shock waves have been spent which still leaves a margin of 400-800 shock waves for additional treatment of areas where the stone appears to be not sufficiently fragmented.
Case 3 demonstrates this approach in a typical case of a complete staghorn stone in a slightly dilated collecting system (figures 67a-e).

*Case 3:* 34 year old female; 3 previous stone incidents, no stone surgery; history of recurrent urinary tract infections. Previous stone analysis was calcium oxalate monohydrate and the current stone analysis revealed a struvite stone.

Figure 67a shows the complete staghorn stone in a larger than normal, and slightly dilated collecting system extending into all the calices. The radiographic stone density is slightly higher than the density of ribs.

The IVP presented at the initial clinical evaluation showed the course of the ureter to be unremarkable and there was no indication for a stenosis distal to the stone.

This constellation made the patient suitable for ESWL treatment.

In this specific case, the stone responded well to the shock wave treatment (figure 67b). Because of the large stone burden a staged procedure was performed.

Figure 67b shows the situation after the first session of ESWL. During this session 2,000 shock waves at 20 kV were delivered, and all stone parts but those in the upper caliceal group were treated and nicely disintegrated.
Figure 67c shows that prior to the second ESWL session, which was undertaken two days later. At this time most of the stone particles had cleared the collecting system. No major hydronephrosis was detected on ultrasound. A second session was then undertaken at which 2,100 shock waves at 20 kV were delivered to the remaining stone parts.

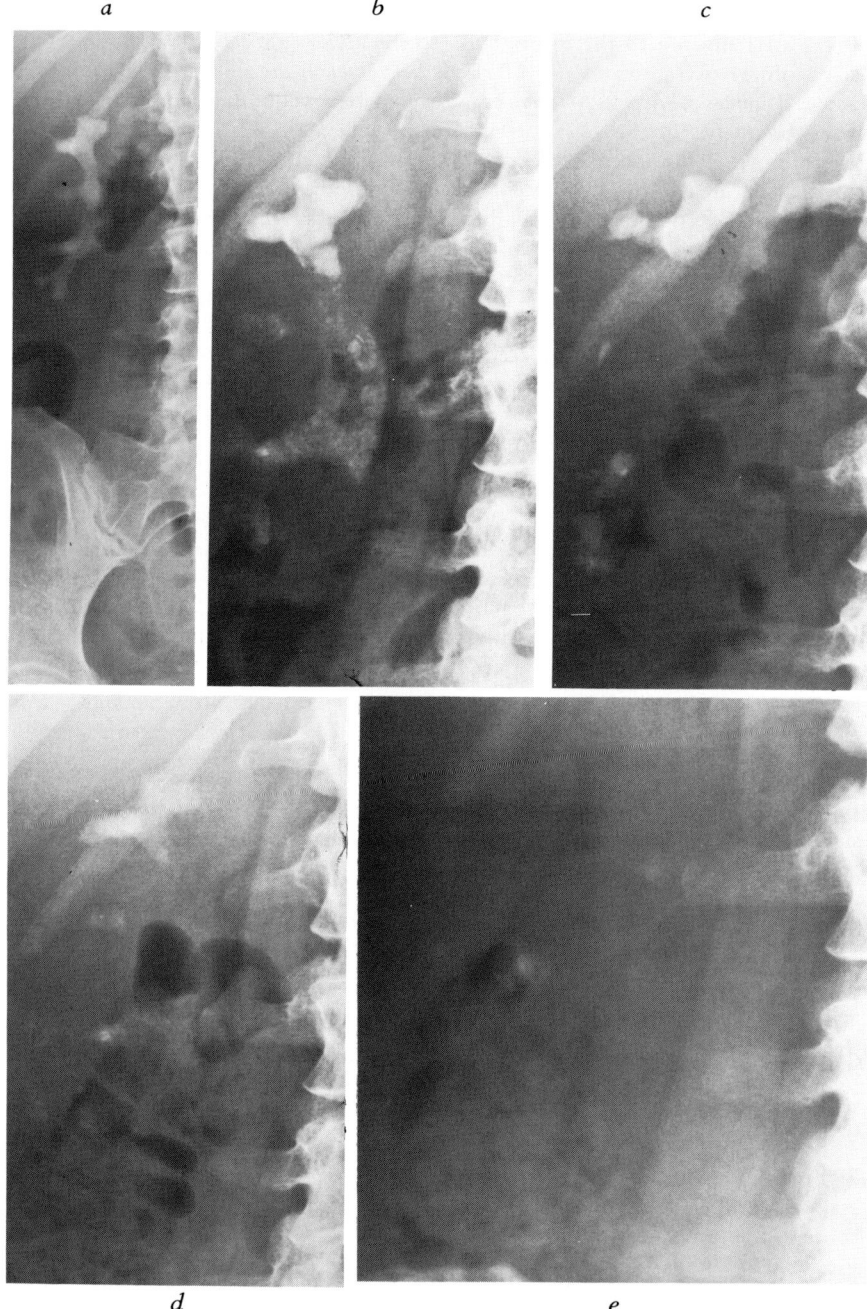

*Figure 67 a-e.* Case 3: ESWL of staghorn stone filling a slightly dilated collecting system.

Figure 67d shows the KUB taken immediately after the second ESWL session confirming the complete disintegration of all stone parts. A KUB taken on post-day 26 (figure 67e) reveals only a few remaining, but by size, spontaneously passable fragments. The patient eventually became stone free after 6 weeks.

c) Treatment of staghorn stones in solitary kidneys

The management of staghorn stones in solitary kidneys deserves special considerations. Because of the large stone burden, and the resulting increased likelihood of ureteral obstruction during the passage of the fragments with consecutive impairment of renal function, these patients have to be closely followed. The fact that the discharge of all fragments may last longer than 3 months, and the relatively high rate of possible complications during this extended period of time actually requires an excellent patient compliance.

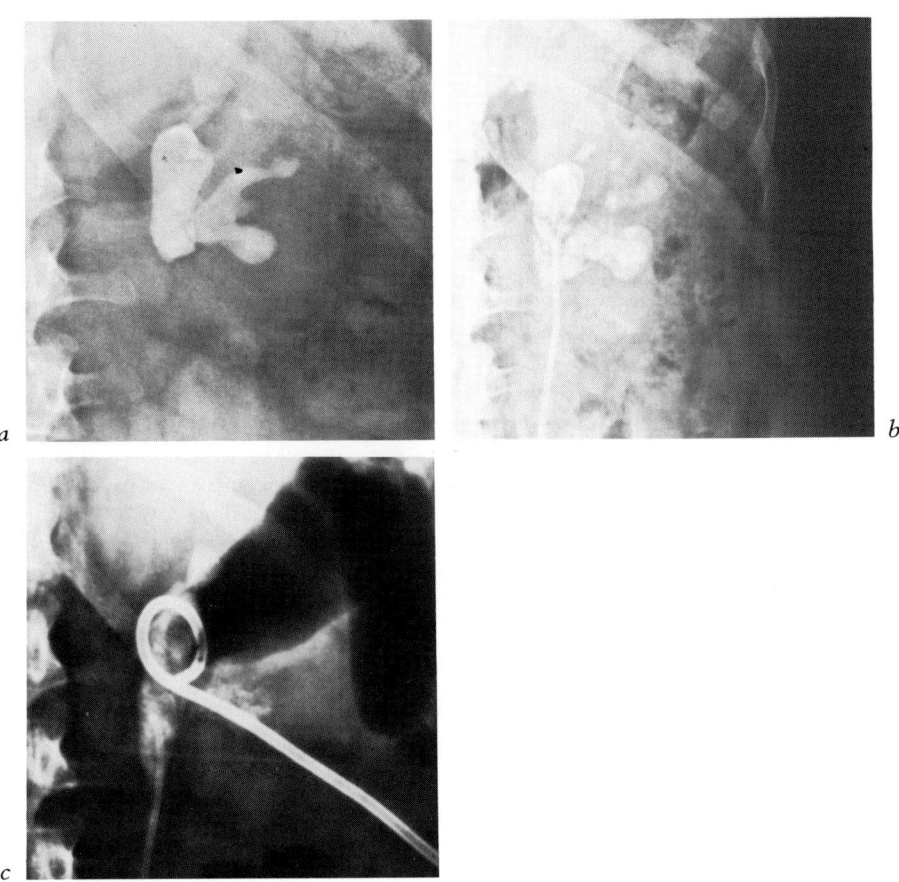

*Figure 68 a-c.* Case 4: ESWL of staghorn stone in a solitary kidney.

Figure 68a-c depicts the steps in the management of a large partial staghorn stone in a dilated collecting system, in a patient with a solitary kidney.

*Case 4:* 41 year old female; two previous stone surgeries on the left side; right nephrectomy for a urosepsis secondary to obstructive stone disease. The stone analysis of the present stone revealed 60 % struvite and 40 % calcium oxalate monohydrate. Pre-op creatinine was in the range of 2.8 mval/l, and post-operatively at the 3-months follow-up it was 1.7 mval/l.

Patients with increased creatinine levels are usually evaluated with a retrograde pyelogram prior to treatment. In this case, the patient brought the respective films with her which showed the ureter to be patent and revealed no subpelvic or intrarenal obstruction. This made this patient eligible for ESWL treatment, and after a two day i.v. antibiotic treatment of her urinary tract infection, ESWL treatment ensued as a staged procedure.

Figure 68a shows the large staghorn stone in a dilated collecting system. The stone density is slightly higher than that of a rib.

During the first session of ESWL 2,400 shock waves at 20 kV were delivered to the stone parts in the pelvis, and mid and lower caliceal group.

Figure 68b shows the complete disintegration of the treated stone parts after the first session of ESWL. At this time a double-J stent was inserted to prevent migration of larger remaining stone parts down into the ureter.

This procedure is actually performed in all staghorn stones where the impression after the first session indicates that stone parts in the range of up to 4 mm remain, which eventually could pass into the ureter and therefore would require ureteral manipulation prior to the following session. In patients with a solitary kidney who undergo a staged procedure, double-J stent placement is mandatory in most of the cases to prevent the hazard of immediate ureter blockage by larger stone particles.

The immediate follow-up in this particular case was then rather stormy. Despite adequate antibiotic coverage, the patient spiked a high fever due to obstructive pyelonephritis. This actually necessitated placement of a percutaneous nephrostomy tube on post-day 1 after the 1st session. Owing to the drainage by the nephrostomy tube, and antibiotic coverage, the symptoms resolved quickly so that the 2nd session was performed 4 days later. At this time 1,600 shock waves at 20 kV were delivered to the remaining stone parts leading to complete disintegration of all stone parts (figure 68c). Further follow-up was unremarkable and all fragments were discharged within 11 weeks.

Whenever required, in patients with solitary kidneys the nephrostomy tube is usually left indwelling during the entire period of stone passage.

When there is only a small percentage of up to 10 % of disintegrated stone material left, the nephrostomy tube is clamped unless the patient develops obstructive symptoms. The tube will be kept closed until eradication of all stone fragments. During the entire period of stone passage, and thereafter for six more months the patient is kept under antibacterial agents.

In principle, fractionated disintegration in 2 or more sessions might be feasible in most cases of staghorn stones filling a non- or mildly dilated collecting system. Because of the large stone deposit, however, the period until the patient becomes stone free is considerably prolonged [5, 9, 10, 12, 23].

Generally, multiple sessions are required to completely disintegrate those stones, and there is a higher incidence for the need of post-ESWL auxiliary procedures. After the ESWL treatment close patient surveillance is necessary to prevent the possible hazards of urosepsis secondary to prolonged obstructive pyelonephritis [5, 9, 10].

This asks for a good patient compliance especially when the patient has to be followed on an out-patient basis for quite a long time.

d) Treatment of staghorn stones filling a grossly dilated RCS

Appreciating this, in staghorn stones with a really large stone mass in an enlarged RCS (equal to or greater hydronephrosis grade II), a percutaneous procedure is performed first for debulking the stone to reduce the stone mass. In a second session, usually after 2 to 4 days, ESWL is employed for the remaining caliceal stone parts.
Depending on the size of the original stone three or more sessions, either percutaneous nephrolithotomy (PCN) under local anesthesia or additional ESWL treatment under epidural anesthesia have to be undertaken (figure 69, table X). This combined approach is now routinely used for the treatment of excessively large stones [9-12].

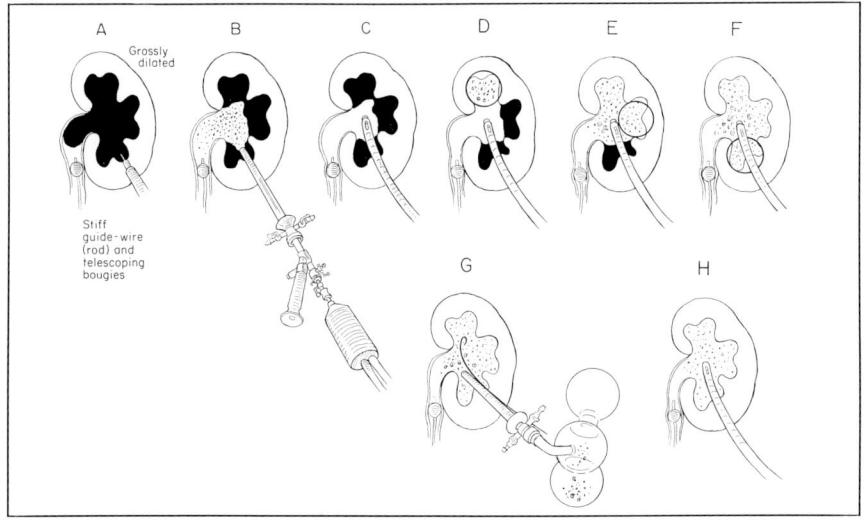

*Figure 69.*   Schematic drawing; technique of the combined treatment of debulking PCN and ESWL.

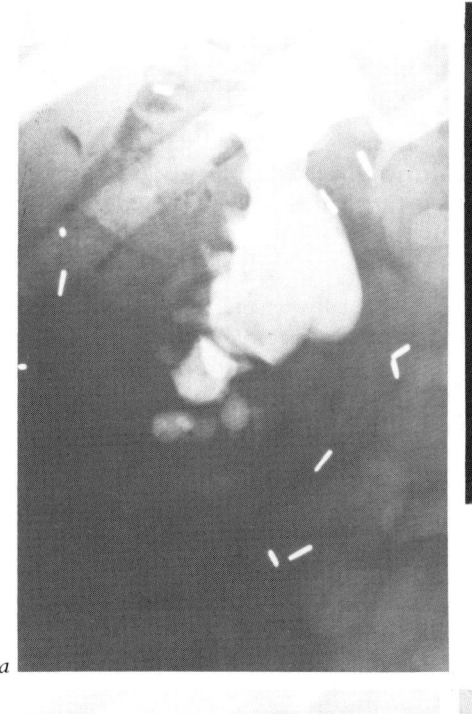
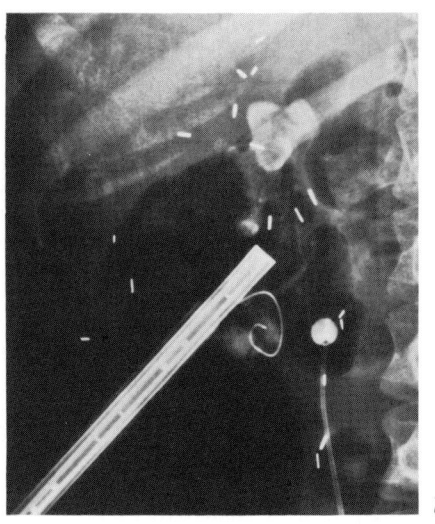
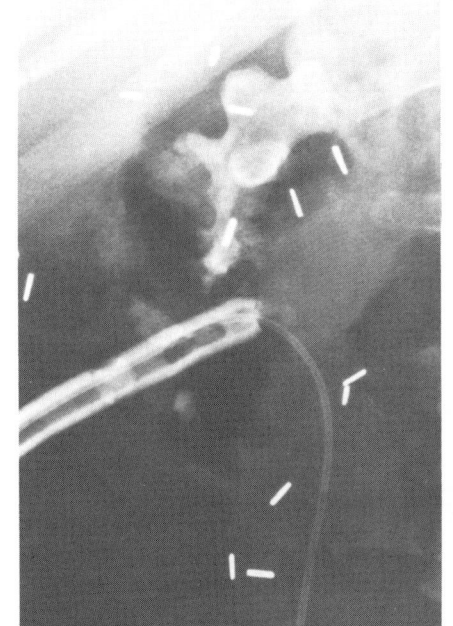
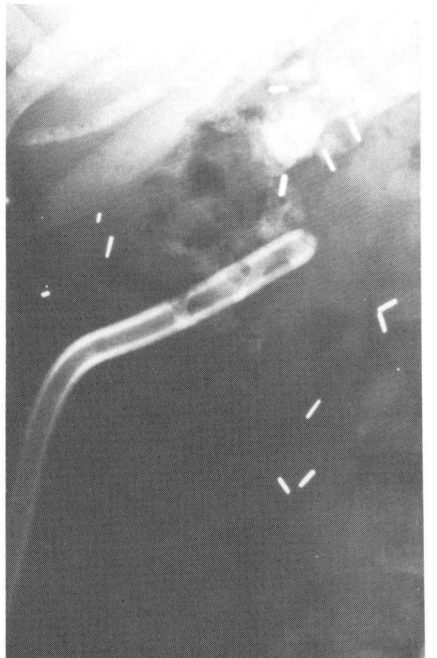

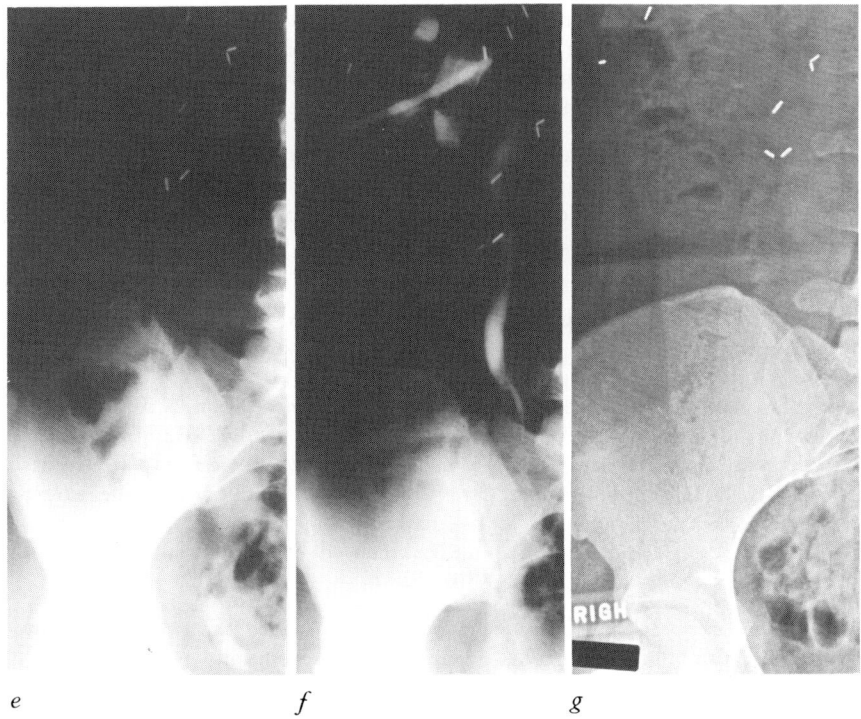

*e*  *f*  *g*

*Figure 70 a-g.* Case 5: Treatment course of PCN and ESWL in the treatment of a staghorn stone filling a grossly dilated RCS.

*Tactical approach:* After establishment of a percutaneous tract through a lower pole posterior calyx, a one stage percutaneous nephrolithotomy is performed. Due to the fact that the access calyx is completely cast out by stone material in most cases, it is usually not possible to place a guidewire about the stone. For this reason the percutaneous access is negotiated, and the track secured during dilation, by poking the stiff end of the Lunderquist-guidewire into the stone. The track is then dilated up to 24 Fr. using the Alken telescoping bougies. This has to be performed very carefully under repeated fluoroscopic control. Over the last bougie the 26 Fr. nephroscope sheath is passed and advanced to the stone. Then the optical insert and the ultrasound transducer are introduced and moved onto the stone [9-11]. Removal of the stone part in the lower calyx and advancing the nephroscope accordingly, helps to secure the track and to prevent losing of the track which would be difficult to renegotiate due to the lack of a safety guidewire, and the fact that in a one stage procedure no mature tract exists [10].

Optionally, ESWL to the lower calices can be performed in a first session. This facilitates the passage of a safety guide-wire for the ensuing percutaneous procedure [5-7]. The percutaneous procedure, however, should not be performed in the same session as a considerable amount of bleeding may be encountered. Two days after the initial session the resulting hyperemia in the treated area has usually been resolved, and the percutaneous approach can be performed in the regular one-stage fashion.

During the percutaneous session (1st session in the combined approach; 2nd session when ESWL was performed first), all stone material which can be easily reached from one percutaneous track is removed. At the conclusion of this session, a 24 Fr. nephrostomy tube secures the urine drainage from the kidney (figure 69c).

After the hematuria resulting from the percutaneous stone surgery has subsided, ESWL is employed for the remaining caliceal stone parts. This is usually undertaken 3-4 days after the percutaneous procedure [10]. Up to 2,000 shock waves at an average of 21 kV are delivered during one session. A 3-4 day pause between the sessions of percutaneous treatment, and ESWL treatment is strictly obeyed in all cases. The reason for this is the previous experience with one of the early combination cases where ESWL followed stone surgery immediately, and fragmented stone material migrated into the parenchyma through lesions of the intrarenal mucosa caused by the initial percutaneous procedure.

After extracorporeal shock wave lithotripsy has led to the complete disintegration of the remaining stone particles, these eventually pass through the nephrostomy tube as well as down the ureter (figure 69). Those particles in the ureter, however, constitute no special problem as urine drainage is secured by the nephrostomy tube. Depending on the size of the original stone, additional sessions with percutaneous stone surgery or ESWL may be indicated. In the case of a large amount of disintegrated stone fragments, evacuation of fragments using the Ellik evacuator may be preferred as it allows for quick eradication of the debris [9, 10].

Depending on the individual patient, all the different steps in the combined treatment of staghorn stones can be undertaken under epidural catheter anesthesia. In the patient with a low compliance, however, general anesthesia for the initial percutaneous procedure should be preferred [9, 10].

Case 5 gives an example for the management of a complete staghorn stone filling a grossly dilated collecting system (figure 70).

*Case 5:* 18 year old female; two previous open surgeries for recurrent stones on the right side; history of recurrent urinary tract infections. The previous and the present stone analysis was calcium oxalate monohydrate.

Figure 70a shows a complete staghorn stone in a grossly dilated collecting system with a stone density higher than that of rib.

The IVP provided for evalutation showed no stenosis distal to the stone. She was then accepted for treatment and initially a one-stage percutaneous stone removal was performed under general anesthesia.

Figure 70b shows the situation at the conclusion of the first session with most of the stone parts in the lower caliceal group, all stone parts in the renal pelvis and some of the upper caliceal group removed.

The KUB (figure 70c, d) was taken prior to ESWL treatment, which was performed three days after the PCN. At that time, 2,100 shock waves at an average of 21 kV were delivered to the remaining stone particles leading to complete disintegration of all stone parts (figure 70d, e). Post-operatively the patient did well, most of the stone fragments passed without problems through the nephrostomy tube and down the ureter. After five weeks the patient accidentally lost the nephrostomy tube, and due to ureteral obstruction leading to urine drainage from the percutaneous entry site replacement of the nephrostomy tube was indicated (figure 70e, f).

Two weeks later, a second session of ESWL was performed for fragmentation of remaining fragments in the mid and lower caliceal group which measured up to 4 mm. In this session 1,400 shock waves at an average of 20 kV were delivered. Postday-3 KUB shows that the patient was stone free days after the second ESWL procedure (figure 70f, g). At this time the nephrostomy tube, which was clamped after the second ESWL procedure, could be withdrawn after a nephrostogram was found unremarkable. The patient became stone free after 9 weeks.

e) Results of ESWL treatment of staghorn stones

The results obtained with staged ESWL procedures in the treatment of staghorn stones which fill a non- or slightly dilated collecting system indicate that regarding the high success rate, and the relatively low rate of complications this has become a useful method of approaching these stones [9, 14].

Over the initial three months period after treatment only 64 % of patients with partial staghorn stones, and 58 % patients with complete staghorn stone become completely stone free. The respective figures after 6 months, however, are 77 % and 70 % which is almost as good as in stones of up to 2.5 cm overall stone mass. Fragments of a size allowing spontaneous passage remain in 19 % and 23 %, respectively, and larger particles indicating additional ESWL treatment are found in 4 % and 7 %,respectively (table XV).

Initial treatment of these large stones requires multiple sessions in the majority of cases (63 % partial staghorns, 90 % in complete staghorn stones).

The necessity for percutaneous tube placement to relieve obstruction, and prevent obstructive pyelonephritis is directly related to the original stone size and is considerably higher in larger stones. In partial staghorn stones, 39 % of the patients require percutaneous nephrostomy tube placement, and in the complete staghorn stones 63 % of those cases who had ESWL alone required percutaneous nephrostomy tube placement (9 Fr. or 12 Fr.) at any time during follow-up (table XV).

*Table XV.* Results of treatment of Staghorn stones

|  | Partial | Complete |
|---|---|---|
| *Methods used* | | |
| ESWL | 96 % | 30 % |
| PCN | 2 % | 7 % |
| PCN and ESWL | 2 % | 60 % |
| Surgery | 0 % | 3 % |
| *Stone free* | | |
| At 3 months | 64 % | 58 % |
| At 6 months | 77 % | 70 % |
| *Spontaneously passable* | 19 % | 23 % |
| *Fragments >4 mm:* | 4 % | 7 % |
| *Number of sessions* | | |
| 1 session | 37 % | 10 % |
| 2 sessions | 45 % | 68 % |
| > 2 sessions | 18 % | 32 % |
| *Auxiliary measures* | | |
| PNS-placement | 39 % | 63 % |

The overall invasiveness of the treatment, however, is low and compared with percutaneous stone surgery alone or open surgery, patients tolerate the discomfort from the percutaneous nephrostomy tube well. Usually most patients can resume their work within a couple of days after hospital discharge.

Review of the insertion time of the percutaneous nephrostomy tube indicates that most (75 %) of the nephrostomy tubes are required during the hospital stay. Secondary hospitalizations are required in 8 % of cases. In those cases tube placement is commonly required because of pain associated with fever and gross hydronephrosis. 17 % of nephrostomy tubes were placed in an outpatient setting, as the patients presented with a longer standing but other than this, asymptomatic obstruction.

The duration of percutaneous nephrostomy tube drainage was between 2 days and 5 months, with an average of 20 days.

Manipulation of an extended ureteral "Steinstrasse", is being undertaken less frequently. For one, it is a tedious and time consuming procedure requiring anesthesia and hospitalization in most cases; and secondly, experience has shown that when a percutaneous nephrostomy tube is used more liberally, most patients eventually pass their stone fragments in a natural way. This finding is somewhat astonishing as the back pressure from the kidney is missing when the urine is diverted.

The combination of PCN and ESWL has special advantages in two patient groups with staghorn stones. In the treatment of large staghorn stones filling grossly dilated RCSs, the advantages of a percutaneous debulking procedure are obvious. Though initially more invasive than ESWL monotherapy, the benefits of the planned combined approach are the controllable treatment course, less postoperative complications in regard to obstructive pyelonephritis, and a considerably shortened follow-up until the patient becomes stone free [9, 10, 14].

In the patient with a staghorn stone in a slightly enlarged RCS, the combination is preferable in those cases where the radiographic stone density is notably higher than rib density. Experience has shown that those stones are hard to be managed with two ESWL sessions with an increased likelihood of larger chunks remaining, and a higher rate of auxiliary measures needed to eradicate the incompletely disintegrated particles.

### 5.4.3 Treatment of ureteral stones

Ureteral stones located in the bony pelvis are not primarily amenable to ESWL treatment because most of the delivered energy is absorbed by the bone, or the stones can not be positioned in the second focal point.
Ureteral stones located above the iliac crest, which cause symptoms and are too large to be passed spontaneously, are primarily eligible for ESWL treatment. Initially, ureteral stones were treated in situ with a primary success rate not higher than 50 % [3, 5, 12, 15, 21]. At the time of percutaneous stone removal, or open surgery following unsuccessful ESWL it was found that most of the stones had been fairly well disintegrated though [9, 51, 21]. They could not pass, however, because they were wedged in the edematous ureteral wall. This finding occurred mainly in stones totally obstructing the ureter which were situated at the same place for a period longer than 6 weeks [3-5, 15, 21].

The following depicts the course of an upper ureteral stone treated successfully in situ in the ureter with one session of ESWL.

*Case 6:* 46 year old male; no previous stone history, a stone history was established, indicating that both stones were located in the ureter for approximately 2 weeks prior to treatment. Because of the radiographic appearance of a sufficient expansion chamber, ESWL in situ treatment deemed appropriate.

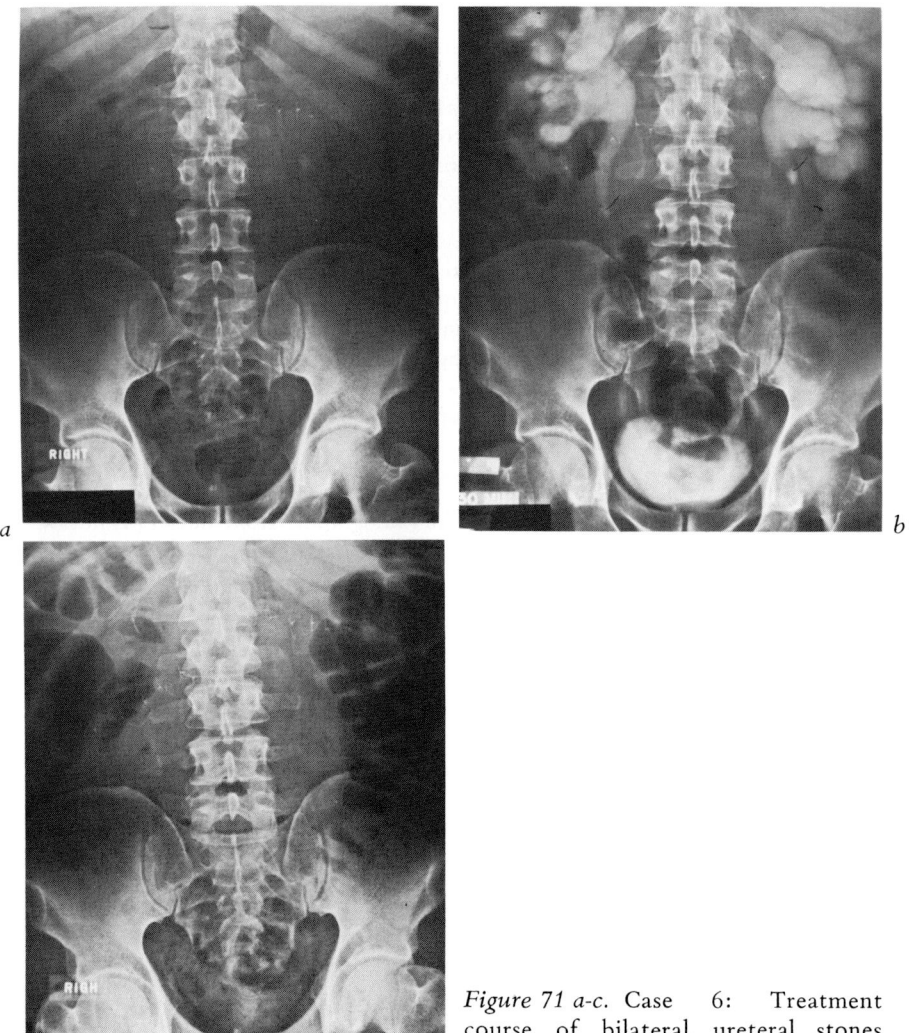

*Figure 71 a-c.* Case 6: Treatment course of bilateral ureteral stones treated with ESWL in situ.

Figure 71a shows the obstructing stones at the level of L4 on the right and at the level of L3 on the left. Figure 71b shows gross hydronephrosis bilaterally, but the contrast dye flows easily along side the stones and no ureteral narrowing is demonstrated. Figure 71c depicts the situation on postday 1. At this time the patient had already become stone free after disintegration was achieved with 1,900 shock waves at an average of 22 kV on the right side on with 1,700 shock waves at an average of 22 kV on the left.

Experience showed that in situ treatment of ureteral stones with a history longer than 6 weeks resulted in a high percentage in only fragmentation of the outer shell of the stone. This, however, will allow subsequent successful stone manipulation. With repeat ESWL sessions and ureteral manipulation, the success rate finally was in the range of 80 – 85 % [9, 12, 15, 21].

Figure 72 depicts a case with a 6 month impacted stone (figure 72a).

*Case 7:* 52 year old female, one previous stone episode.

After manipulation and while placing the Foley catheter into the bladder, the catheter slid below the stone (figure 72c). The stone was treated in the situ (1,600 shock waves at an average of 23 kV) with poor results. Seven days later a second stone manipulation was done (figure 72d), followed by ESWL (1,400 shock waves at 22 kV).

This resulted in complete stone disintegration (figure 72e) and the patient became stone free within 3 days.

Looking further into the causes for failures, it was found that disintegration of ureteral stones is dependent upon the physical contact between the calculus and the ureteral wall. When the ureteral wall is in close proximity to the calculus it means that the stone is wedged in an edematous stone bed. In this case insufficient disintegration will occur because no expansion space is available for stone fragmentation. This finding is regardless of the amount of energy delivered. Therefore, it was believed that successful disintegration of ureteral stones by ESWL is dependent upon the presence of an expansion chamber [13, 18].

For all ureteral stones this can be achieved by two means: relocating the stone into the renal pelvis which constitutes the ideal (case 8, figure 73), or relocating the stone in a ureteral segment amenable to ESWL treatment, i.e., mid or upper ureter, with creation of an artificial expansion chamber of at least 6 Fr. in size (case 9, figure 74).

In most instances, stones which are wedged in the ureteral wall cannot be relocated by "plain" advancement of a ureteral catheter [9, 13, 15, 18, 21]. The latter abuts on the stone as the stone is closely trapped in an edematous stone bed not leaving enough space for the advancement of a ureteral catheter or even a guide-wire. More forceful maneuvers should not be undertaken as they may easily result in ureteral perforation. To facilitate the stone repos-

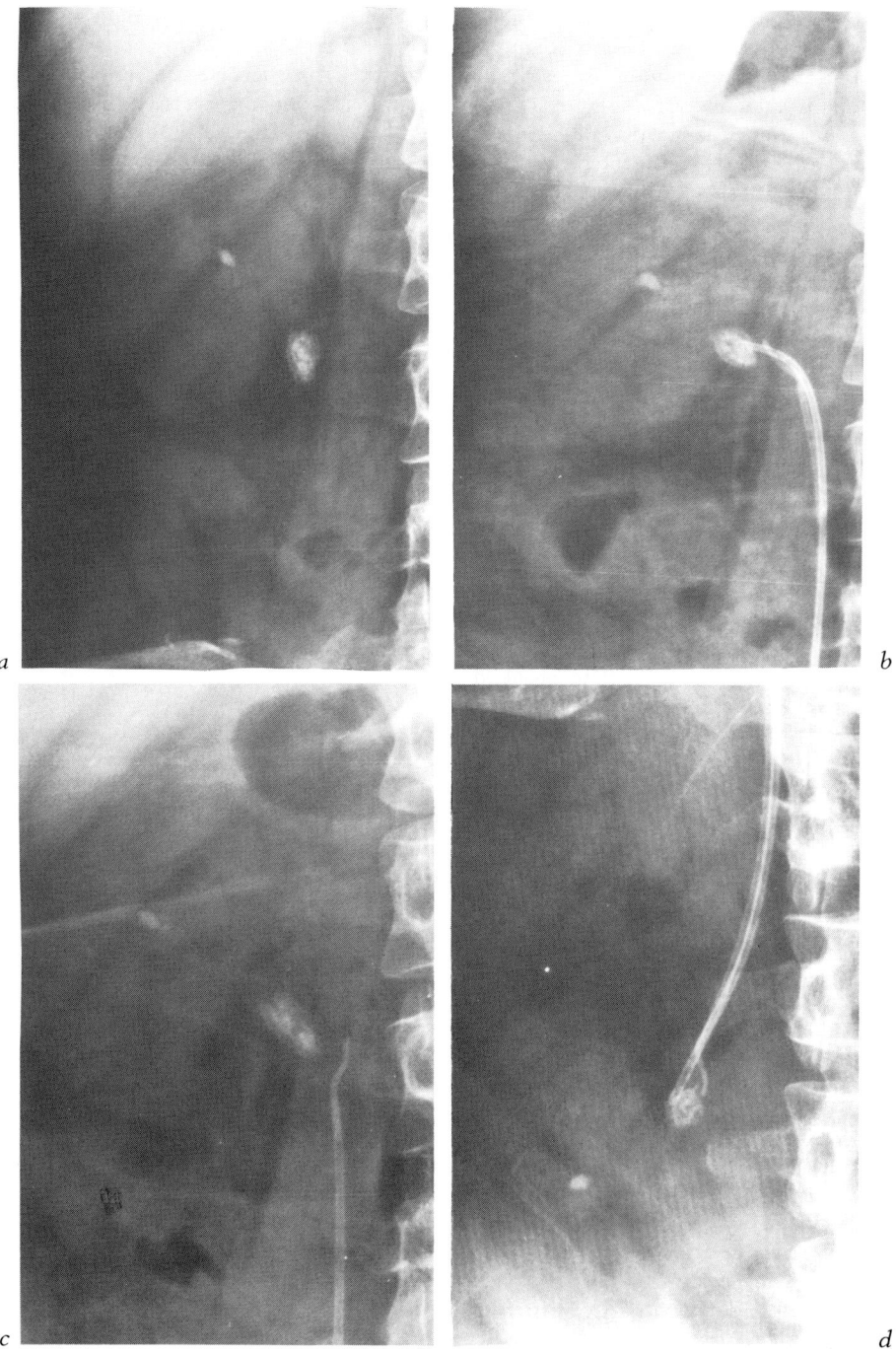

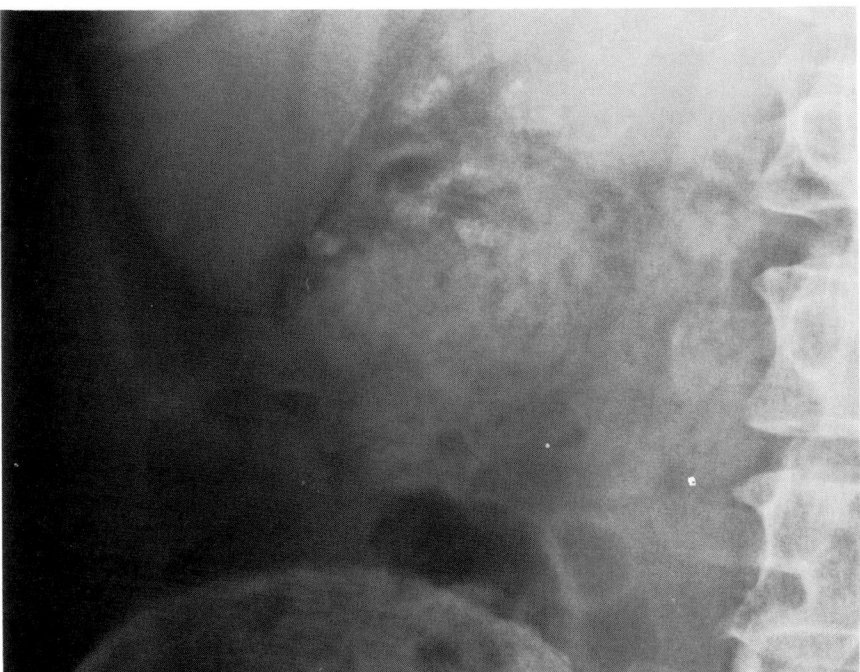

*Figure 72 a-e.* Case 7: Treatment course of ureteral stone treated with ESWL after stone manipulation.

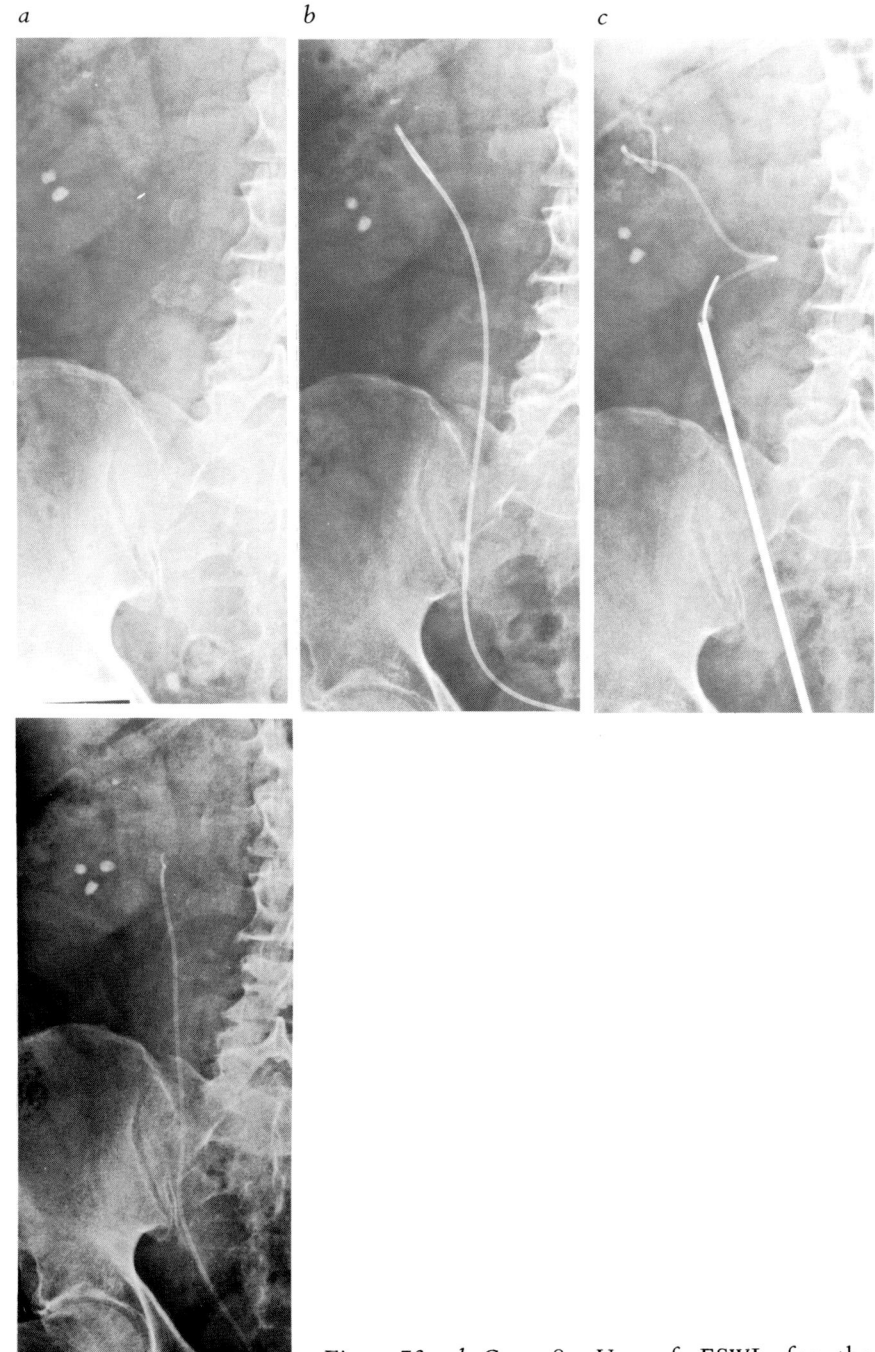

*Figure 73 a-d.* Case 8: Use of ESWL for the treatment of a lower ureteral stone.

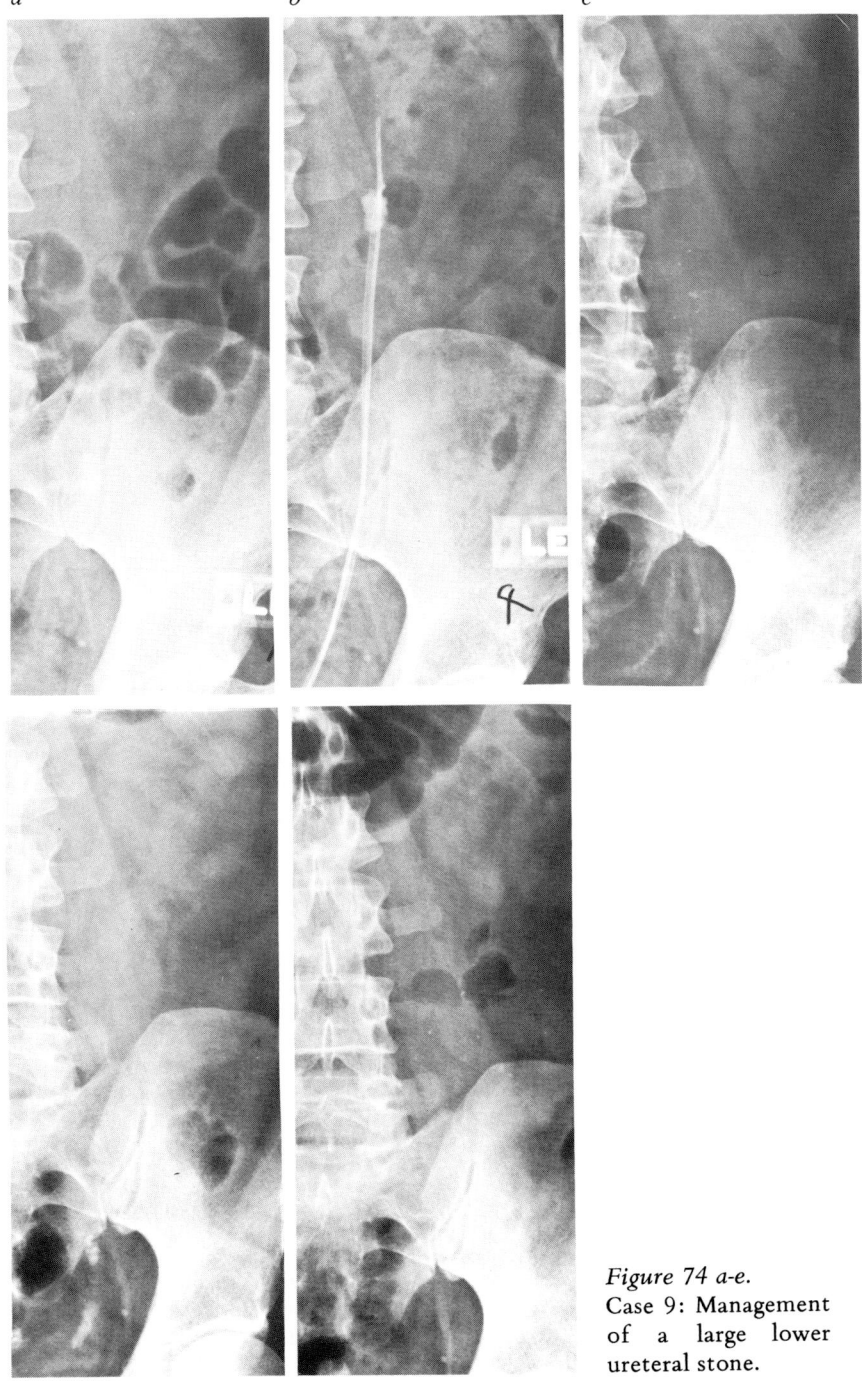

*Figure 74 a-e.*
Case 9: Management of a large lower ureteral stone.

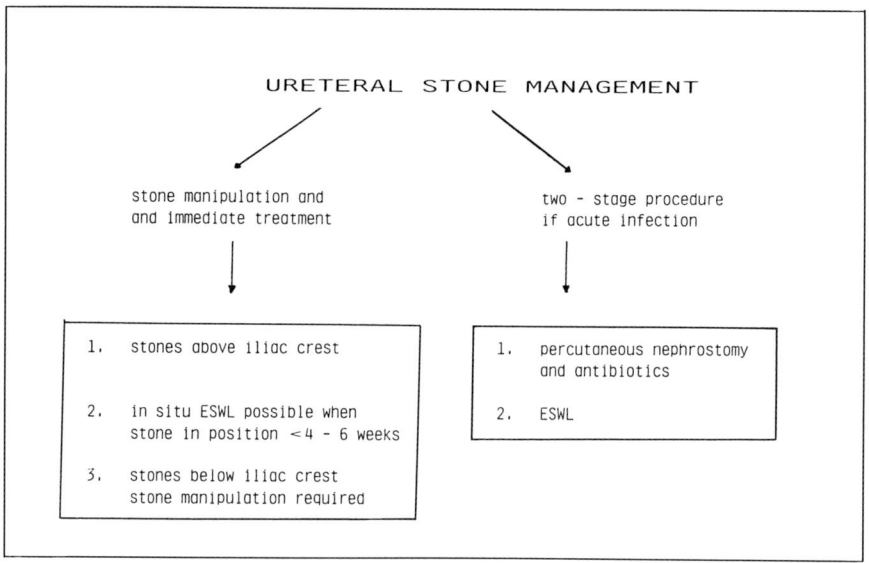

*Figure 75.* Tactical and technical considerations in ureteral stone management.

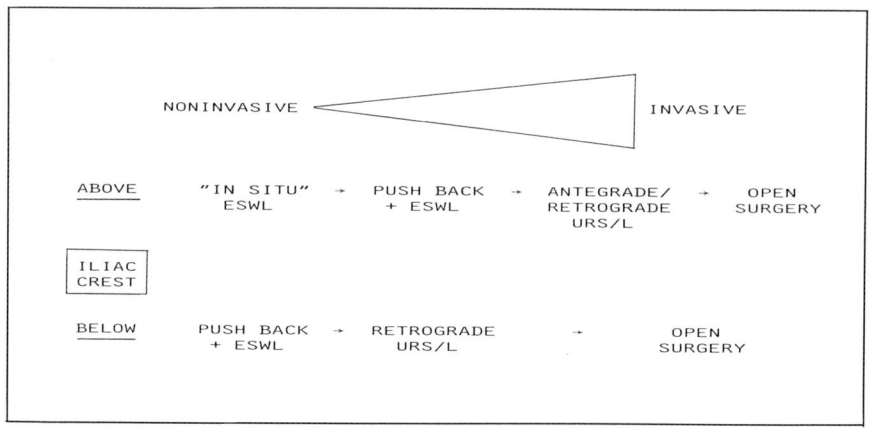

*Figure 76.* Stages of invasiveness in the treatment of ureteral stones.

itioning maneuvers using ureteral lubrication has been found advantageous [13, 18].

Ureteral lubrication is achieved using 2 % water soluble xylocaine jelly admixed to normal saline or destilled water. The proportion of jelly to solvent is such that the solution flows easily when injected into a 6 Fr. ureteral catheter. In general, the admixture represents 20 – 30 % of the jelly to 70 – 80 % solvent.

It takes a few minutes of thorough stirring to obtain good dispersion of solute into solvent. A 6 Fr. or 8 Fr. Braash catheter is advanced to the level of the stone. Five to ten cm$^3$ of solution are forcefully injected, and the stone is "probed" by advancing and retracting the scope and the catheter as a unit for a few millimeters. In most instances, this maneuver is sufficient to displace the stone and relocate it into the renal collecting system (figure 76) [10, 13, 18].

*Case 8:* This is 72 year old male patient with a relatively large stone located in the right terminal ureter, and two stones in the right lower calyx (figure 73a). Passage of a #8 Braash and a #6 spiral tip catheter failed to reposition the stone above the iliac crest (figure 73b). Ureteroscopic stone extraction was then attempted but the stone was too large to be engaged in the basket. The stone was then successfully relocated into the renal pelvis from where it fell into the lower calyx (figures 73c, d).
ESWL treatment with 1,500 shock waves was performed and the patient became stone free after 3 weeks.

In cases where the stone cannot be repositoned into the renal pelvis a different approach is followed. The aim of the procedure is to position the stone in a ureteral segment accessible to ESWL, or in the renal pelvis. When the stone is located or repositioned in the mid or upper ureter and can not be advanced into the renal pelvis, the aim is to create an expansion chamber of at least 6 Fr. in size for successful ESWL disintegration [13, 18].

To create an expansion chamber an aray of catheter combinations is employed, such as 5 Fr. whistle tip and 6 Fr. spiral tip, two #4 spiral tip catheter a.s.o. When possible, a 6 Fr. spiral catheter is advanced along-side the Braash catheter to the level of the stone. Lubrication and stone "probing" is repeated several times. When the spiral tip catheter passes the stone it is advanced into the renal pelvis, and the Braash catheter is left below the stone to prevent migration of the stone. The catheter(s) is then securely attached to a 14 Fr. or 16 Fr. Foley catheter left indwelling in the bladder [13, 18].

Even unusually large stones located in the lower ureter can be relocated and successfully treated.

*Case 9:* This 25/16 mm stone is obviously too large for endoscopic extraction and its location precludes primary ESWL treatment (figure 74a). Using a #6 Fr. spiral tip and a #5 whistle tip catheter, the stone was repositioned in the mid ureter with the #5 Fr. whistle tip which was passed along-side the stone, and the #6 Fr. spiral catheter below the stone (figure 74b). ESWL treatment was successful with 1,800 shock waves at 22 kV (figure 74c). On postday 1 a "Steinstrasse" is seen in the terminal ureter (figure 74d) and on the next day the patient was already stone free (figure 74e).

When the ureteral stone is completely impassable, placement of a 6 Fr. spiral tip catheter may prove helpful. The tip of the catheter inserts itself between the stone and the ureteral wall, and the spiral part of the catheter cups itself under the stone thus creating an expansion chamber [13, 18].

When the stone cannot be retrogradely manipulated at all with ureteral stents, ureteroscopic extraction or repositioning is employed as the next step. If this can not be achieved ultrasonic disintegration through the ureteroscope is performed [9, 13, 15, 18, 21] (figure 76).

a) Results of ESWL treatment of ureteral stones

Using the above mentioned regimen results in a success rate of 96.6 %. The remainder can be rendered stonefree with the use of the ureteroscope [13]. Open surgery has become the exception and is only employed when all the other methods have failed, or when indicated to correct anatomical alterations at the time of stone removal (figure 76). It can be anticipated that most of the patients treated successfully with this combined approach will need one session of ESWL (95.5 %) [13].

In most cases stone manipulation is performed in a retrograde fashion. The antegrade route is chosen when the distal ureter is not readily accessible due to a supravesicular urinary diversion, or when a percutaneous access already exists and the stone is located in the upper 2/3 of the ureter [13].

Whenever the stone(s) can not be repositioned, an attempt is made to pass a ureteral catheter along-side the stone to create an artificial expansion chamber (table XVI) [13, 18].

The success rate of those patients whose stones are repositioned into the renal collecting system does not differ from stones of similar size treated initially in the kidney (table XVIII) [13]. The amount of necessary energy is similar to that used for native stones in the kidney. This seems to indicate that an

*Table XVI.* Methods used to manipulate ureteral stones prior to ESWL

| Pre-ESWL | |
| --- | --- |
| Ureteral catheter | 89.4 % |
| Ureteroscopic repositioning | 2.0 % |
| Overall success rate of pre-ESWL stone manipulation | 91.4 % |
| Alternative methods applied (after failed UC-manipulation or in situ ESWL) | |
| Ureteroscopic extraction | 2.5 % |
| Ureteroscopic ultrasound lithotripsy | 6.1 % |

Table XVII. Results of pre-ESWL stone manipulation and success rates

|  | % | Success disintegration | Stone free at 2 wks/3 mts | |
|---|---|---|---|---|
| Ureteral stones repositioned into renal coll. system (RCS) | 59 % | 100 % | 85 % | 98 % |
| Upper ureter + stent | 27 % | 94.6 % | 92 % | 99 % |
| Mid ureter + stent | 7.5 % | 91.2 % | 89 % | 99 % |
| Upper ureter no stent | 4.4 % | 48 % | 46 % | * 100 % |
| Mid ureter no stent | 2.1 % | 60 % | 56 % | * 100 % |

* stone free after auxiliary procedures

Table XVIII. Number of shock waves and energy used in relation to stone position at treatment

|  | Success disintegration | Average # of SW | Average kV | Range kV |
|---|---|---|---|---|
| Ureteral stones repositioned in the RCS | 100 % | 1,360 | 20.0 | 19 – 21 |
| Upper ureter + stent | 94.6 % | 1,620 | 22.4 | 21 – 23 |
| Mid ureter + stent | 91.2 % | 1,710 | 22.2 | 21 – 23 |
| Upper ureter no stent | 48 % | 1,900 | 23.4 | 22 – 24 |
| Mid ureter no stent | 56 % | 1,880 | 23.0 | 22 – 24 |

expansion space is the most important variable in the ESWL treatment of ureteral stones, and that the other factors previously incremented, such as mucoid lining, play only a minor role [13].

When treated in the upper ureter, or in the mid third of the ureter above the iliac crest, a success rate almost as high as for stones relocated into the RCS can be achieved once a stent is passed about the stone. The figures are 94.6 % and 91.2 %, respectively (tables XVII, XVIII) [13]. As seen in table XVIII, 3, greater energies than on the kidneys are required for successful disintegration when stones are treated in the ureter in the presence of an adequate expansion chamber. For stones in this location, we advocate the use of $23 - 24$ kV [13].

The success rate drops sharply in those cases where completely obstructing stones with a history of more than 6 weeks are treated in situ in the ureter. Single ESWL treatment is only successful in approximately $50\% - 60\%$ of the cases.

Thus, the convincingly high success rates have made the combined approach the preferred procedure for stones located in the mid or upper ureter, or for any ureteral stone in the distal 1/3 associated to ipsilateral upper collecting system stones [13, 18].

### 5.4.4 Treatment of infected stones

Urinary tract infection is a key consideration in the management of stone disease. Treatment of infected stone patients is no longer a contraindication for ESWL. Clear indications and guidelines for therapeutic and prophylactic antibiotic use have been established.

Experience has shown that patients with existing urinary tract infections can be safely treated with ESWL once appropriate antibiotic treatment is initiated at least 24 h prior to ESWL treatment. ESWL therapy results in fragmentation and dispersement of stone material, during this process possibly liberating bacteria from the infected stone core in cases of infected stones. So this possibility has to be considered in patients with a history of urinary tract infection, and no existing urinary tract infection at the time of treatment. According to the experience gained over the years, ESWL patients are categorized into four groups:

Group I: patients without history of infection, a negative urinalysis at admission, and negative urine culture.

Group II: patients without history of infection, a positive urinalysis at admission, and negative culture.

Group III: patients with history of infection, positive urinalysis at admission, and negative culture.

Group IV: patients with history of infection, positive urinalysis at admission, and positive culture.

For better practicability and to reduce the hospital stay, patients with a history of infection are pre-screened by their referring urologist one week prior to admission, and antibiotic therapy is initiated as needed. In patients without history of infection, a urine sample is collected upon admission, and urinalysis and urine cultures are performed.

Approximately 25 % of ESWL patients fall into category I and are considered a low risk to experience post-treatment pyelonephritis.

Without administration of a prophylactic antibiotic, however, the percentage of up to 25 % of post-operative fever episodes was surprisingly high, which led us to the conclusion that a prophylactic antibiotic should be administered. In our institution it is now a common practice to administer one dose of a cephalosporine on-call to the ESWL unit. This regimen has tremendously reduced the occurrence of post-ESWL pyelonephritis in this patient group and now the incidence runs below 6 %.

Most patients, that is 45 %, fall into category II which places them at a higher risk than those in group I. These patients also receive prophylactically one dose of a cephalosporine. Under this regimen only 9 % of patients were found to run a post treatment temperature of greater than 38.5 °C.

21 % of patients fall into group III which places them at a considerably high risk of harboring infected stone nidi. To prevent post ESWL pyelonephritis antibiotic treatment is installed 24 h prior to ESWL and is continued for 48 h. Under this regimen 98 % of patients remained free of temperature after ESWL.

4 % of patients had active infections at the time of hospital admission. These patients had the antibiotic treatment installed 24 h prior to treatment and they remained on antibiotics for at least 5 days after ESWL. Under this regimen also 98 % of patients remained asymptomatic with regard to postop temperature.

This regimen shows that deliberate use of antibiotics based on the patient's history and the present laboratory findings can greatly reduce the risks of post-ESWL obstructive pyelonephritis and this way most infection stones and infected stones can receive ESWL treatment. The only exception to this rule is in patients presenting with obstructing ureteral stones and associated infection. In those cases a percutaneous nephrostomy tube is placed first and antibiotic treatment is installed. Once the symptoms have subsided ESWL treatment is performed according to the guidelines explained in chapter 5.4.3.

### 5.4.5  Treatment of radiolucent and semi-opaque stones

Radiolucent and semi-opaque stones, such as uric acid stones, certain cystine stones and faintly visible struvite stones, are not primary indications for ESWL as they can not be readily localized with the X-ray system [3-9, 11, 12, 14, 23].

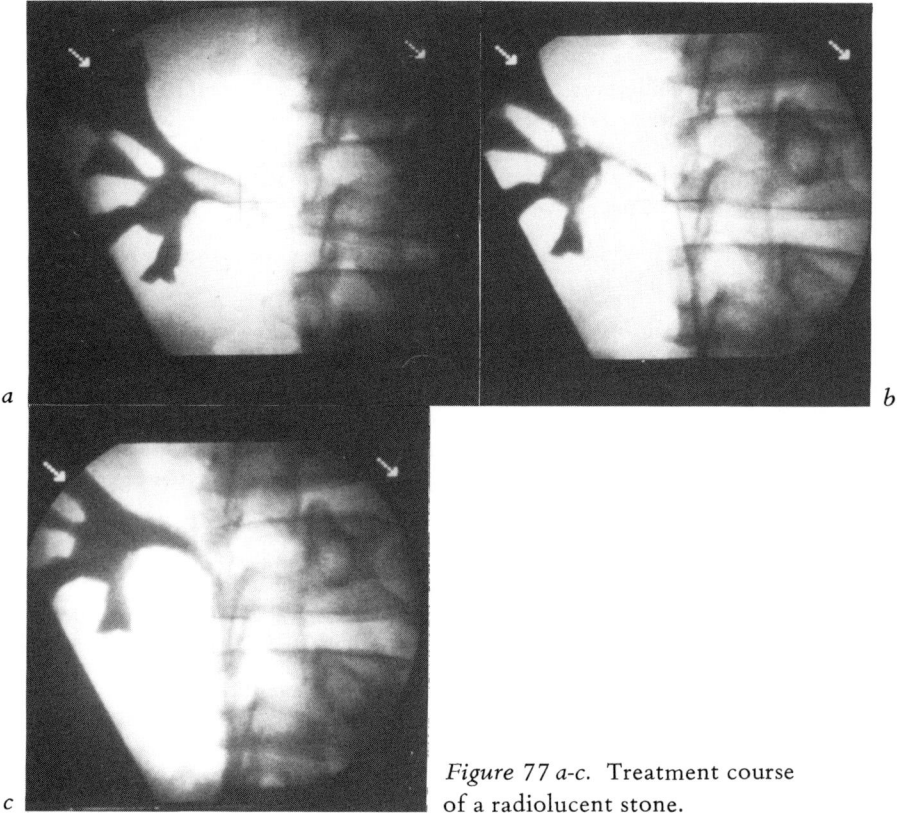

*Figure 77 a-c.* Treatment course of a radiolucent stone.

X-ray visualization of radiolucent and many semi-opaque stones is only possible after administration of contrast medium. Therefore, cystoscopy is performed prior to ESWL under the same anesthesia and a ureteral stent passed up to the ureteropelvic junction. Then contrast dye is injected as necessary, and the stone can be localized with the X-ray systems by aiming on the filling defect (figure 77a). Proper assessment of the degree of disintegration, however, is difficult. With increasing fragmentation, the pre-existing filling defect will usually wane and finally the contrast dye will outline the entire collecting system (figure 77b, c).

In many cases, a clear cut decision as to when fragmentation of the stone is sufficient cannot be easily obtained, and treatment is arbitrarily terminated based on experience with previous cases with similar stones. The same problems are commonly encountered, when performing a diagnostic retrograde pyelogram immediately before ESWL treatment, so that this should be performed in a separate session or the collecting system has to be thoroughly rinsed prior to ESWL. Radiolucency of the disintegrated stone material also hampers the follow-up examinations as the degree of stone disintegration and location of the debris can only be obtained with ultrasound (table XIII) [9].

### 5.4.6 Treatment of bilateral stones

Bilateral stone disease is found in approximately 10 % of our stone patients.

With the availability of a noninvasive treatment modality also the approach to bilateral stone disease has undergone a change. Other than in conventional and endourological surgery ESWL as a noninvasive procedure does not necessitate a second interventional procedure for treatment of contralateral stones. From a technical standpoint ESWL of bilateral stones can be performed under the same anesthesia in the same session after repositioning the patient.

Understandably, the currently symptomatic stone should be treated first. In the presence of a contralateral renal stone, not symptomatic at the time of treatment, simultaneous treatment can be justified under several conditions. One reason is that the procedure is noninvasive by its nature, has a low complication rate and may eradicate the stone before it becomes more troublesome either by increasing size, infection, or by dropping into the ureter requiring additional procedures.

However, no additional risk for the patient should result from this bilateral treatment. Thus, based on experience with renal stones the stone size related complication rates determine the limiting factors. The present guidelines exclude the following stones for simultaneous treatment:

1. contralateral stones, larger than the symptomatic stone,
2. stones in the presence of urinary tract infection or stones suggesting infection-induced origin by radiological appearance.

In order to not increase the risks of post-procedural complications the contralateral stone should be less than 8 mm in size and the necessary number of shock waves anticipated for successful disintegration less than 1,000.

In the rare case of bilateral ureteral stones the symptomatic stone is treated only and in a second session after complete eradication of the stone material the contralateral stone is approached. If a contralateral ureteral stone is found at the time of evaluation for a symptomatic stone in the opposite kidney, the obstructing stone is approached first and the further treatment plan follows the above guidelines.

### 5.4.7 Treatment of children

In most countries nephrolithiasis involving the upper urinary tract is a relatively rare incident in the pediatric age group. The underlying cause in the majority of pediatric stones in the upper urinary tract is a metabolic disorder, in most cases resulting in a high recurrence rate. For this reason the advent of a noninvasive treatment modality for children was especially appreciated.

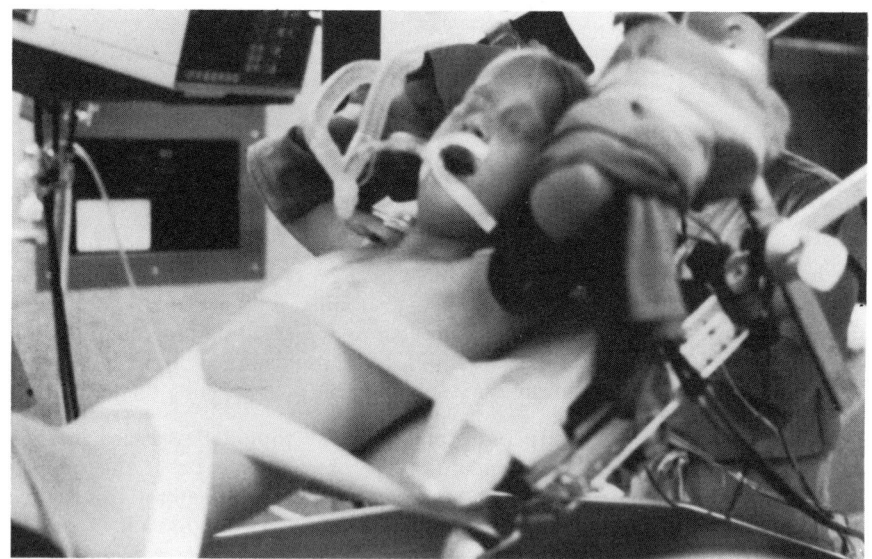

*Figure 78.* Treatment of children.

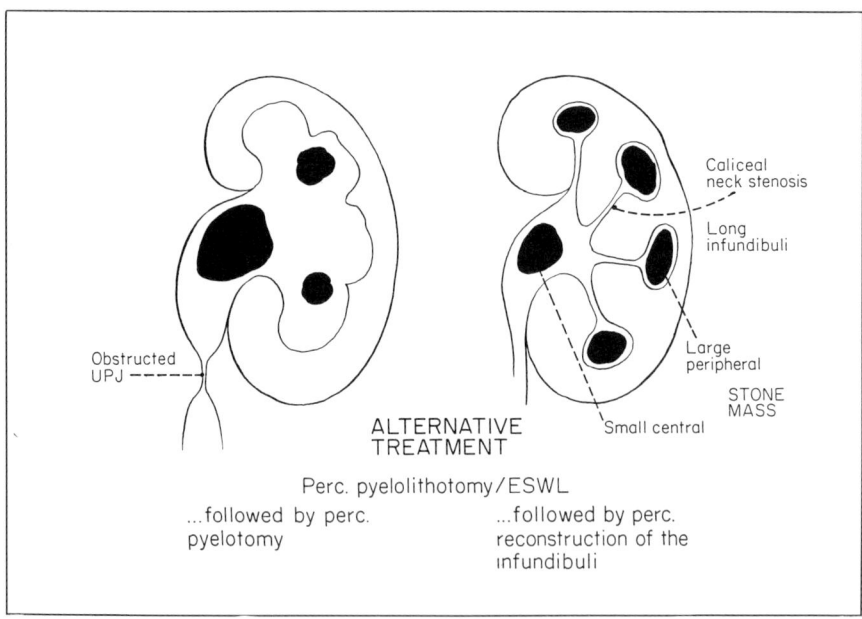

*Figure 79.* Remaining indications for open surgery.

ESWL is particularly advantageous as it can be repeated, as necessary, without detrimental adverse effects to the kidney function [3-9, 11, 12, 23].

With the Dornier lithotripter currently available, children not smaller than 120 cm can receive ESWL treatment. Smaller children cannot be positioned on the patient support [3, 9, 11, 23].

Because of the close proximity of the pediatric kidney to the lung area special measures to protect the lung tissue have to be undertaken. To prevent the lungs from being hit by the shock waves, a styrofoam layer is positioned in the back of the little patient to cover the lower region of the lungs. A radiodense wire attached to the caudal border of the styrofoam allows exact positioning of the protective cover (figure 78).

Treatment is performed under general anesthesia to ensure that the child does not move during the procedure, and to keep the respiration movements low — a further prophylaxis of lung exposure. The energy used is less than in adults, and usually 15 kV to 19 kV suffice to disintegrate most stones with the exception of some cystine stones.

In general, children eliminate the disintegrated stone material faster and with less problems (pain, pyelonephritis) than adults with stones of similar size.

*5.4.8 Treatment of medical risk group patients*

Two medical risk groups deserve special attention: the patient with the corrected coagulopathia (5.4.3.a) and cardiovascular risk patients.

Most cardiovascular risk patients, i.e., patients with hypertension or a heart condition can receive ESWL treatment at major medical centers where appropriate care and follow-up surveillance is available [5-9, 11, 12, 20]. These patients are treated under general anesthesia which allows close monitoring of the cardiocirculatory and lung parameters (ECG, BP, CVP, PWP). Analysis of the Munich patient group according to the risk group grading of the American Association of Anesthesiologists shows that 4.9 % of the patients which were successfully treated belonged to ASA group 4, that means they were cardiopulmonary high risk patients (table XIX).

*Table XIX.* ASA-risk group distribution of ESWL-patients

|  | Risk group | | | | |
|---|---|---|---|---|---|
|  | I | II | III | IV | V |
| % Patients | 40.91 | 37.80 | 17.00 | 4.29 | 0 |

## 5.4.9 Treatment of stones with distal obstruction

Severe narrowing at any level of the urinary tract (caliceal neck, UPJ, ureter, ureteral orifice, BPH, urethral stricture) with secondary distension of the collecting system which is not attributable to the stone itself often precludes successful ESWL treatment [3, 9-12, 23]. Though sufficient stone disintegration can be achieved in most cases, ESWL should not be considered as the primary therapy because of possible problems with the discharge of the fragmented particles. In these cases, either surgical repair of the alteration or a percutaneous procedure are preferable. Of course, either of these can be reasonably combined with ESWL when indicated by a stone location unfavorable for these methods.

Relative obstruction not attributable to the stone does not necessarily rule out the successful use of ESWL. If the stone becomes symptomatic with intermittent pain at the time of excessive fluid charging with quick resolution thereafter, ESWL is the preferred method [9, 10].

Patients with upper urinary tract stones amenable to ESWL treatment, and prostatic enlargement with a residual urine volume in excess of 100 cc should undergo prostatic surgery prior to ESWL [9].

Primary indications for open surgery are stone cases requiring repair of totally obstructing UPJ-stenosis. In these cases, all stone parts which can be reached from the renal pelvis are removed at the time of correction of the underlying obstruction. Approximately 5 – 8 days postoperatively, the UPJ-anastomosis has healed and when a nephrostogram reveals no extravasation, ESWL can be safely performed for the remaining caliceal stone parts (figure 79) [8, 12, 23].

This combined approach allows for removal of complicated staghorn stones with minimal trauma to the parenchyma as caliceal stone fragments formerly accessible only by nephrotomies can be readily disintegrated by ESWL [9-12].

## 5.4.10 Treatment of the "inoperable" stone

Its noninvasiveness and proven absence of any adverse long-term effects on kidney function soon established ESWL as a most beneficial therapeutic tool in the treatment of those patients whose stone and kidney situation precluded any other surgical procedure except nephrectomy. After successful treatments were performed on more than 200 selected patients, the Munich group began to accept patients whose status could be best described as hopeless regards the amount of deterioration of kidney function, number of previous surgeries on the kidney, and the present stone situation.
Attempts at treating those patients with ESWL were undertaken in order to prevent those patients from slipping into terminal renal insufficency or to try to wean them off of hemodialysis. It was soon shown that there indeed was a possibility to successfully treat at least the obstructing stone parts and preserve

and improve valuable residual kidney function. Prerequisite for successful elimination of disintegrated stone material is a water diuresis in excess of 1.5 l per day.

*Case 10:* A 52 year old male patient with nephrocalcinosis. He had a 20 year history of continuous stone passages and six surgical procedures on both kidneys. His right kidney was nonfunctioning and during a bout with obstructive pyelonephritis, he slipped into renal failure requiring temporary hemodialysis. At this time, a percutaneous nephrostomy tube was inserted and his kidney function slowly improved. After decompression and antibiotic treatment, the serum creatinine went back to between 5 and 6 mg/dl. It was decided to treat the obstructing stones in the ureter, renal pelvis, and the calices with ESWL.

Figure 80a: KUB of the patient at the time when he was being treated with hemodialysis. It shows a tremendous amount of calcifications in both the renal parenchyma and the renal collecting system bilaterally. As the left kidney was his functional, solitary kidney, a percutaneous nephrostomy tube was inserted to relieve the obstruction.

Figure 80b shows the situation after the first treatment with ESWL. At this time the stone parts in the ureter and part of the stones contained in the renal pelvis were treated. Figure 80c depicts the situation three days after this session, the first session of ESWL, and shows a deposit "Steinstrasse" in the terminal ureter.

Figure 80d shows the situation after a second session of ESWL was performed for those stone parts of whom it was assumed that they were in the renal collecting system.

Six weeks after initiation of ESWL therapy the renal function had dramatically improved, and after a nephrostogram had demonstrated patency of the ureter, the nephrostomy tube was withdrawn, and the patient was no longer in the need of hemodialysis (figure 80e).

## 5.5  Results of ESWL therapy

The initial results of the first three years, when the lithotripter was only operational in Munich, indicated the high success rate and proved the absence of any long-term adverse effects on kidney function [5-7].

During this period 1,000 patients successfully underwent ESWL treatment for a rate of 90 % of patients, who were found stonefree at a three month follow-up. In 9.3 %, disintegrated and by size spontaneously passable fragments were found and in 0.7 %, of patients surgical procedures to relieve longer standing ureteral obstruction were performed [5-7].

Comparison of these results with the overall Munich results of the last six years, also including the more complex stones which were later accepted, delineates the importance of the original stone size and also the impact of the transport capacity of the upper urinary tract (table XX).

*Table XX.* Results of ESWL treatment (worldwide)

|  | Munich | Stuttgart | Sapporo | UCLA |
|---|---|---|---|---|
| *Date of opening* | 2/80 | 10/83 | 9/84 | 3/85 |
| *Success rate* | 99.0 % | 99.1 % | 99.0 % | 99.5 % |
| *Stone free* (at 3 months) | 84 % | 85 % | 77 % | 80 % |
| Spont. passable | 11 % | 11 % | 19 % | 16 % |
| Fragments > 4 mm | 4 % | 4 % | 3 % | 4 % |
| Open surgery | 1 % | 0.2 % | 0.5 % | 0 % |
| *Complications* | | | | |
| Fever | 6 % | 3 % | 5 % | 4 % |
| Pain/colic | 25 % | 28 % | 32 % | 22 % |
| *Auxiliary measures* | 16.4 % | 17.6 % | 15.8 % | 19.0 % |
| Pre-ESWL | 5.1 % | 10.3 % | 4.4 % | 12.2 % |
| Post-ESWL | 11.3 % | 7.3 % | 11.4 % | 6.8 % |

Very soon the outstandingly good results of the Munich group were reproduced by the Stuttgart group, the second center to receive the lithotripter human model #3 [12].

Comparing our most recent learning curve free results at UCLA with the two first centers, and Sapporo the first ESWL center in Asia, impressively endorses the safety, reliability and reproducibility of the ESWL method (table XX).

### 5.5.1 Renal function

Split renal function studies using J-131 hippurane showed no alteration of renal function over a 4 year period.
Incidentally, the renal function which was set at 100 % prior to ESWL increased after treatment as is shown on the graph (figure 81). This increase is explained by the number of cases where obstructive stones have been treated successfully, resulting in improvement of renal function [3-7].

## 5.5.2 Complications of ESWL and management of ESWL-related complications

Complications from the shock wave treatment itself are extremely rare.

Due to careful medical evaluation and proper patient preparation, anesthesiological complications during the treatment are also rarely seen.

Table XXI depicts the possibilities of intra-procedural complications and their management. In our experience the incident for intra-procedural complications was less than 1 %, necessitating termination of treatment in less than 0.5 % of cases.

All of our patients have been, and are routinely checked with ultrasound for exclusion of damage to the kidney and adjacent organs (table XIII). In our personal experience only 16 out of 5,000 patients (2,200 in Munich, 1,800 in Stuttgart and 1,000 at UCLA) developed a perirenal hematoma. This was suspected by the routine ultrasound and/or clinical symptoms and the diagnosis finally confirmed with CAT scan studies.

Most of those cases have in common a treated blood clotting defect, or one which was not detected with routine laboratory tests (PT, PTT, platelet count, bleeding time). All of them were over 40 years of age, most of them over 60 years. Reasons for the bleedings were partly of vascular origin, and partly qualitative platelet abnormalities in patients having ingested aspirin prior to

*Table XXI.* Management of complications occurring during ESWL

— Close monitoring by anesthesiologist
  (BP, ECG, CVP, AP, PWP)

  — appropriate medication and balanced fluid intake

— Termination of treatment

  in BP problems not responding to medication

  in absolute arrhythmia

— Stone not disintegrated: second session/alternative procedure

— Parenchymal edema: minimal after adequate pre-op hydration

| | | |
|---|---|---|
| BP | = | blood pressure |
| ECG | = | electrocardiogram |
| CVP | = | central vein pressure |
| AP | = | arterial pressure |
| PWP | = | pulmonary wedge pressure |

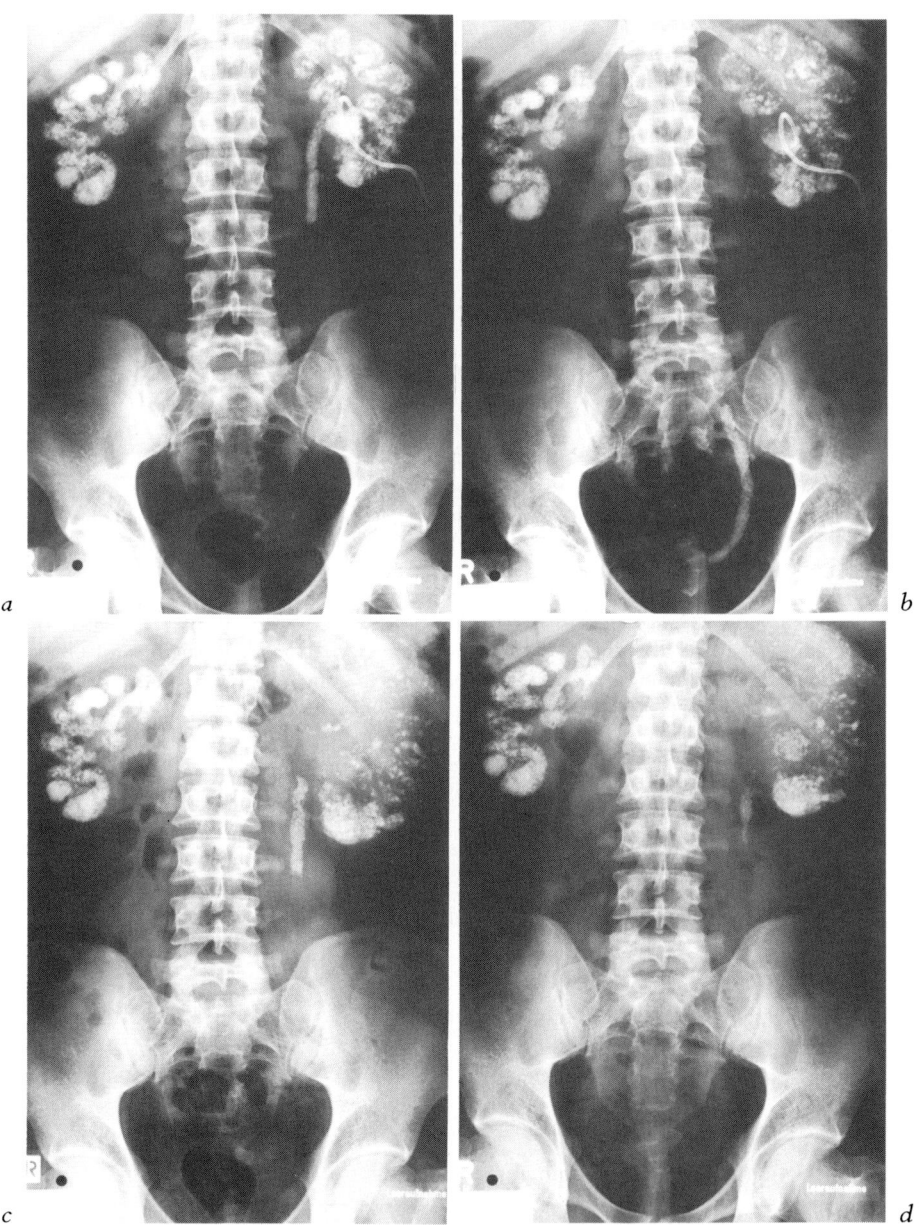

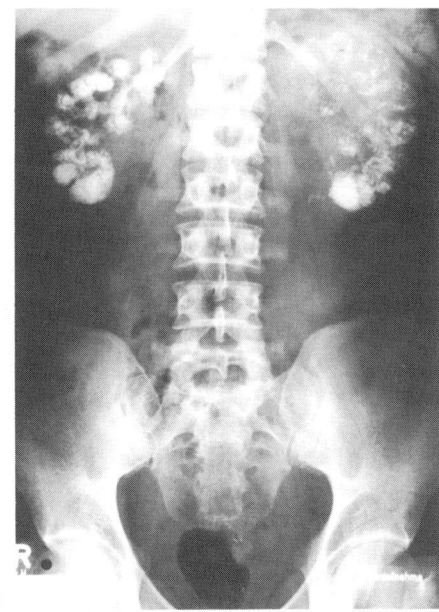

e

*Figure 80 a-e.* ESWL treatment of inoperable stone.

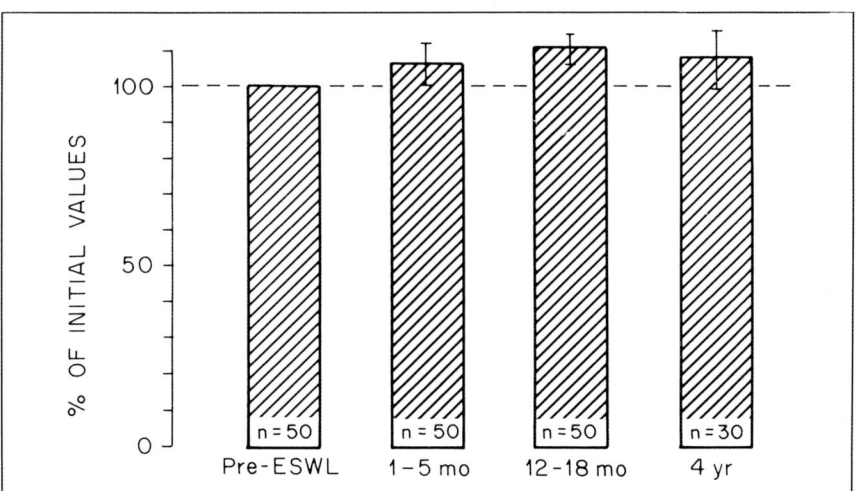

*Figure 81.* Renal function after ESWL.

ESWL treatment. For this reason, aspirin or acetylsalicyl-acid containing medication should be discontinued at least 7 days before the scheduled treatment. Even when normal or marginal clotting parameters are demonstrated, treatment should be deferred whenever aspirin or similar drugs were taken as platelets are sensitive to very low doses of aspirin.

*Table XII.* Management of perirenal bleeding after ESWL

| Perirenal bleeding | |
| --- | --- |
| Diagnosis US, CT, LAB | |
| Blood pressure stable | Blood pressure instable |
| Conservative management "Watchful waiting" | transfusion surgery |

In all cases no significant intrarenal hematoma was ever seen.

All of the cases could be managed conservatively with close observation of blood pressure, central venous pressure and the pertinent laboratory data. Only 50 % of those patients needed blood transfusion and the amount of blood administered was between 2 and 12 pints, and averaged 3.2 pints.

No permanent sequelae of perirenal bleeding remained. All patients had normal CAT scan studies after 6 – 12 months, and no high blood pressure developed in any of the patients. The renal function as determined by creatinine values and hippurane clearances returned to normal within 6 months in all cases.

Given the high acceptance of risk group patients, the rate of ESWL complications is surprisingly low. This is best appreciated by the careful patient preparation we strictly adhere to. How this can be achieved with a similar patient group on an out-patient basis remains unclear to the authors.
Post-ESWL complications include insufficient stone disintegration, and during the passage of the fragments obstructive symptoms such as pain and obstructive pyelonephritis.

Insufficient stone disintegration mainly depends on the size of the original stone, its hardness, location and its radiographic density (table XXI).

With sufficient experience the outcome of the ESWL procedure in terms of stone disintegration can be very well predicted, and the respective guidelines are outlined in chapter 5.4 of this book. Following these guidelines more than 95 % of all stones can be treated with ESWL either as a sole therapy (70 – 75 %), or in combination with endourological procedures (20 – 25 %) [5-12, 14, 23] (figure 63).

In most cases of combined treatment the approach is carefully planned, (i.e., staghorn stones, ureteral stones). Usually the endourological procedure is performed first, (i.e. PCN-debulking in staghorn stones, stent or URS manipulation in ureteral stones) [9-12, 14, 23].

*Table XXIII.* Management of post-ESWL ureteral obstruction

*Asymptomatic*

Close control (US, KUB, Crea, BUN; weekly)

Lasting > 4 weeks:

Ureteral manipulation (LOOP, URS, PCN)

*Symptomatic*

(Colic)  medication

(Fever)  nephrostomy tube, antibiotics, ureteral manipulation

---

These planned pre-ESWL procedures with ensuing ESWL have been tested in various series, and the efficacy has been demonstrated. Comparison of the auxiliary procedures performed at various centers shows that the overall figures do not differ greatly, whereas the breakdown into pre- and post-ESWL auxiliary procedure reflects the tactical biases of the different centers (table XX).

Especially in the treatment of approximately 20 % of more complex stones, the ESWL experience and endourological skill of the operator is required to treat those stones with a similarly high success rate in a minimally invasive fashion.

By no means, and this reflects the experience of all major groups using ESWL, should ESWL be performed on non-selected patients without a strong background in endourology. The minimal requirements are percutaneous nephrostomy tube placement, and the ability to perform ureteral stone manipulation with stents and ureteroscopes, if required.

Further post-procedural complications are mainly secondary to ureteral obstruction. Discomfort or pain is found in approximately 25 % of all cases, and half of these patients responds well to oral pain medication, or if nausea co-exists to suppositories.

Owing to the guidelines concerning the deliberate use of periprocedural antibiotics, the incidence of post-ESWL obstructive pyelonephritis is relatively low, and no major difference between the various centers is observed (table XX). Auxiliary procedures after ESWL are mainly indicated when obstructive pyelonephritis has to be relieved to prevent urosepsis. In our service we liberally use percutaneous nephrostomy tube drainage. This together with appropriate antibiotic treatment quickly relieves the acute symptoms, and even in the presence of an extended ureteral "Steinstrasse", the fragments are eliminated within a reasonable period of time (table XXIII).

Appreciating our previous experience with ureteroscopic manipulation of extended Steinstrasse, we do not favor this approach at all. Ureteroscopy for treatment of "Steinstrasse", is a tedious, difficult and highly hazardous undertaking, which should only be performed when a larger piece of debris proceeds the deposit "Steinstrasse" and blocks the ureter. Other than this, plain nephrostomy tube drainage can deal with most of the "Steinstrasse", cases.

In the management of solitary large chunks in the ureter, the same approach as for a native ureteral stone (see 5.4.3) is chosen.

## 5.6 The role of ESWL in current concepts of urinary stone management

ESWL, the noninvasive method of disintegration of upper urinary tract stones has experienced an unprecedented success in the past six years [3-9, 12, 14, 23]. Experience has shown that not all stones behave equally, and the outcome of the procedure was found to be dependent on and influenced by various factors. Treatment success is to a great extent determined by the size of the original stone(s), stone location, and the presence of anatomical and/or functional alterations of the upper urinary tract.
Taking this into account the overall results are broken down into different groups to obtain comparable results.
During the past six years of clinical application, three main groups of ESWL stones have evolved. Accordingly "easy" kidney stones, "complicated" kidney stones, and upper ureteral stones are evaluated separately [9, 10,12].

In all kidney stones, the rate of successful stone disintegration is in the range of 99 % (table XX). Only a small minority of all renal stones, namely cystine stones cannot be successfully fragmented with ESWL. It can by no means be predicted, however, which of these stones will not respond sufficiently [5-8, 12, 23].

Experience has shown that solitary or multiple kidney stones of an overall size of up to 2 cm without obstruction distal to the stone, can be considered "easy" stones for ESWL treatment with regard to the simplicity of treatment, a 99 % success rate, and a low rate of postprocedural complications (tables XX, XXIV).

Coincidentally stones of this size are also considered ideal for percutaneous removal [1, 9, 10, 17, 19, 24, 25]. When planning a percutaneous stone removal, the actual stone location needs special attention, however, as stones located in middle and upper calices are more difficult to approach percutaneously [1, 9, 10, 17, 19, 24, 25].

ESWL offers the advantage that all radiopositive renal stones irrespective of their actual location in the collecting system can be easily localized and treated [3-9, 11, 12, 23]. Considering that 25 % – 35 % of renal stones are located in or extend into the middle and upper calices, shows the clear advantage ESWL has in the treatment of these patients.

*Table XXIV.* Complications after ESWL, comparison of "easy" and "problem" stones

|  | Pain/Colic | Fever | Auxiliary measures |
|---|---|---|---|
| "Easy" stones | 24 % | 5 % | 4 % |
| "Problem" stones | 34 % | 36 % | 35 % |

*Table XXV.* Auxiliary measures after ESWL

|  | Ureteral manipulation | Percentage nephrostomy | Surgery |
|---|---|---|---|
| "Easy" stones | 5 % | 1 % | 0 |
| "Problem" stones | 22 % | 26 % | 2 % |

Thus noninvasiveness, the simplicity of treatment, and the lower rate of postprocedural complications explain why percutaneous stone removal is being increasingly superseded by ESWL in the treatment of the so called "easy" stones [9, 24].
Stone location and configuration of the upper urinary tract mainly influence the choice of treatment.
Considering these factors, approximately 70 % – 80 % of nonselected stones categorize into the group of "easy" stones.

In the remainder various combinations of ESWL with endourological procedures have been tried out and according to the favorable results treatment guidelines have now been established for most upper urinary stones.
Approximately 5 % – 10 % of a nonselected patient group are patients with stones larger than 2.5 cm, partial, and complete staghorn stones.

Experience with ESWL monotherapy of larger stones showed a significant increase in the rate of complications during fragment discharge after successful stone disintegration. This finding is consistent with a relatively high rate of auxiliary procedures needed, and a prolongation of the hospitalization time (tables XXIV, XXV).
Thus the choice of treatment strategy has to be thoroughly considered and each case should be carefully evaluated according to the guidelines explained in chapter 5.4.

Obstruction distal to the stone is one of the major obstacles to successful ESWL treatment. The usual approach in all those cases where no clearcut indication for open surgery can be made is to start with the noninvasive method, ESWL, and wait for the results of the 3 months follow-up.

If at this time the debris has not cleared the kidney a repeat treatment has to be considered. In those cases of disintegrated renal pelvic or caliceal stones with stenosis hampering proper discharge of the fragments, or in stones presenting with severe functional alterations of the motility of the upper urinary tract, the combination of ESWL with a percutaneous procedure has the advantage that the underlying anatomical anomaly can be corrected at the time of percutaneous surgery.

With the advent of ESWL and endourological procedures urinary stone management has changed dramatically. Proper and reasonable use of each of the methods, alone or in combination, has diminished the need for open surgical intervention. To which extent open surgery can be avoided depends mainly on the availability of all treatment modalities (ESWL, PCN, URS) and, of course, on the experience of the urologist. So at the most experienced stone centers more than 97 % of all patients referred are treated without resorting to open surgery [9, 10, 12, 14].

The few indications for open surgery include cases of pediatric stone disease in children smaller than 100 cm where none of the new methods is applicable, and certain patients with severe anatomical anomalies (extreme kyphoscoliosis, spastic contractions, horseshoe kidneys).

Also an indication for open surgery is seen in staghorn stones with a small central, that is pelvic, and a large peripheral, that is a caliceal stone mass, especially when associated with a long, narrow infundibula (figure 79).

In these cases direct removal of the stones through nephrotomies is preferable as the disintegrated particles would not pass through the narrow infundibula [9-12].

The management of urinary stone disease has completely changed in the past five years since the introduction of extracorporeal shock wave lithotripsy as a noninvasive treatment modality. In this period of time ESWL has almost completely surplanted open surgical and to a lesser extent endourological approaches.

The reason for this surprisingly rapid progress with this new methodology is only partially explained by the excellent research cooperation of urologists and physicists. The high demand for a less invasive treatment modality exerted by the stonebearing patients themselves was also a major contributing factor. Therefore the anticipated high exceptations were not met immediately. It was, however, important that the outside pressure did not influence the cautious approach in increasing the indications. Based on the noninvasive concept of the methodology, a stepwise enlargement of the indications backed by reproducible results was pursued, which lead to well established indications for the treatment of all upper urinary stones.

We surely do not know, whether or not we have reached the endpoint of development of this method and its clinical applications for the treatment of urinary stone disease. However, it is certain that this progress made by urologists, for the sake of urology, represents a dramatic change in the management of urinary stones by which invasive approaches have been superseded by noninvasive procedure. From now on all other methods employed for the treatment of urinary stones will have to be judged against the results of this new methodology.

## Literature

1 *Alken, P.; Hutschenreiter, G.; Gunther, R.; Marberger, M.:* Percutaneous stone manipulation. J. Urol. *125*, 463-466 (1981)
2 *Chaussy, C.; Brendel, W.; Schmiedt, E.:* Extracorporeally induced destruction of kidney stones by shock waves. Lancet *13*, 1265-1268 (1980)
3 *Chaussy, C.; Schmiedt, E.; Jocham, D.; Brendel, W.; Forssmann, B.; Walther, W.:* First clinical experience with extracorporeally induced destruction of kidney stones by shock waves. J. Urol. *125*, 417-420 (1981)
4 *Chaussy, C.; Schmiedt, E.; Jocham, D.:* Nonsurgical treatment of renal calculi with shock waves. In: Stones, clinical management of urolithiasis. Eds. Roth, R.A., Finlayson, B., Churchill Livingstone, New York (1983)
5 *Chaussy, C.; Schmiedt, E.:* Shock wave treatment for stones in upper urinary tract. Urol. Clins N. Am. *10*, 743-750 (1983)
6 *Chaussy, C.; Schmiedt, E.:* Extracorporeal shock wave lithotripsy (ESWL). An alternative to open surgery? Urol. Radiol. *6*, 80 (1984)
7 *Chaussy, C.; Schmiedt, E.; Jocham, D.; Schueller, J.; Brandl, H.; Liedl, B.:* Extracorporeal shock wave lithotripsy (ESWL) for treatment of urolithiasis. Urology *5*, 59 (1984)
8 *Chaussy, C.; Fuchs, G.:* World experience with extracorporeal shock wave lithotripsy for the treatment of urinary stones: Assessment of its role after 5 years of clinical use. Endourology Newsletter *1*, 7-9 (1985)
9 *Chaussy, C.; Fuchs, G.:* Extracorporeal shock wave lithotripsy (ESWL) for the treatment of urinary stones. In: Textbook on adult and pediatric urology. Ed. Gillenwater, J., Year Book Publishers, Chicago, (in press, 1986)
10 *Eisenberger, F.; Fuchs, G.; Miller, K.:* Extracorporeal shock wave lithotripsy and endourology: An ideal combination for the treatment of kidney stones. World Journ. *3*, 41-47 (1985)
11 *Fuchs, G.; Miller, K.; Rassweiler, J.:* Alternatives to open surgery for renal calculi: Percutaneous nephrolithotomy and extracorporeal shock wave lithotripsy. In: Klinische und Experimentelle Urologie. Ed. Schilling, W.; Zuckschwerdt, München (1984)
12 *Fuchs, G.; Miller, K.; Rassweiler, J.; Eisenberger, F.:* Extracorporeal shock wave lithotripsy: One-year experience with the Dornier lithotripter. Eur. Urol. *11*, 145 (1985)
13 *Fuchs, G.; Chaussy, C.; Riehle, R.:* The use of ESWL for ureteral stones. In: Principles of extracorporeal shock wave lithotripsy. Eds. Riehle, R., Newmann, D., Livingstone, New York (1986)
14 *Fuchs, G.; Chaussy, C.:* Worldwide experience with, and future concepts of ESWL. In: Principles of extracorporeal shock wave lithotripsy. Eds. Riehle, R., Newmann, D., Livingstone, New York (1986)
15 *Gumpinger, R.; Miller, K.; Fuchs, G.; Eisenberger, F.:* Antegrade ureteroscopy. Eur. Urol. *11*, 199-202 (1985)
16 *Huffmann, J.L.; Bagley, D.H.; Lyon, E.S.:* Transurethral removal of large ureteral and renal pelvic calculi using ureteroscopic ultrasonic lithotripsy. J. Urol. *130*, 31 (1983)
17 *Korth, K.:* Percutaneous renal stone surgery, Springer, Berlin, Heidelberg, New York, Tokyo (1984)

18 *Lupu, A.; Fuchs, G.; Chaussy, C.:* A new approach to ureteral stone manipulation for ESWL. In: Endourology Newsletter *1*, 13 (1985)
19 *Marberger, M.; Stackl, W.; Hruby, W.:* Percutaneous litholapaxy or renal stones. Eur. Urol. *8*, 236-242 (1982)
20 *Miller, K.; Fuchs, G.; Bub, P.; Rassweiler, J.; Eisenberger, F.:* Financial analysis, personnel planning and organizational requirements for the installation of a kidney lithotripsy at an urologic department. Eur. Urol. *2*, 210-217 (1984)
21 *Miller, K.; Fuchs, G.; Rassweiler, J.; Eisenberger, F.:* Treatment of ureteral stone disease: The role of ESWL and endourology. Wld Journ. *3*, 445 (1985)
22 *Perez-Castro Ellendt, E.; Martinez Pineiro, J.A.:* Transurethral ureteroscopy — a current urological procedure. Arch. Esp. Urol. *33*, 445 (1980)
23 *Schmiedt, E.; Chaussy, C.:* Extracorporeal shock wave lithotripsy of kidney and ureteric stones. Urol. Int. *39*, 193-198 (1984)
24 *Segura, J.W.; Patterson, D.E.; Le Roy, A.J.* et al: Percutaneous lithotripsy. J. Urol. *130*, 1051 (1985)
25 *Wickham, J.; Miller, R.:* Percutaneous surgery of renal calculi, Churchill-Livingstone, London (1983)